In the Way of Our Grandmothers

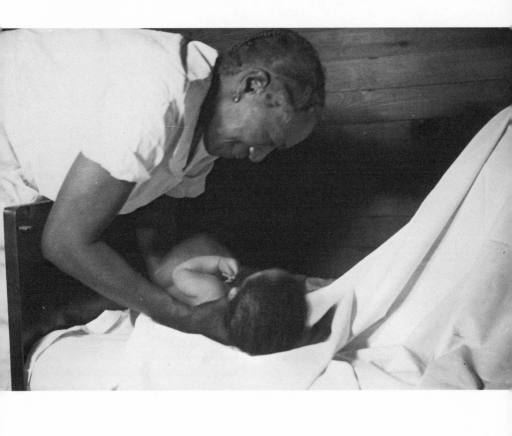

In the Way of Our Grandmothers

A Cultural View of
Twentieth-Century Midwifery
in Florida

Debra Anne Susie

The University of Georgia Press
Athens and London

© 1988 by the University of Georgia Press
Athens, Georgia 30602
All rights reserved

Designed by Kathi L. Dailey
Set in Mergenthaler Sabon
Typeset by The Composing Room of Michigan
Printed and bound by Thomson-Shore, Inc.

All of the photographs in this book are from the Florida State
Archives, Tallahassee.

The paper in this book meets the guidelines for
permanence and durability of the Committee on
Production Guidelines for Book Longevity of the
Council on Library Resources.

Printed in the United States of America

92 91 90 89 88   5 4 3 2 1

Library of Congress Cataloging in Publication Data

Susie, Debra Anne.
   In the way of our grandmothers.

   Includes index.
   1. Midwives—Florida—History—20th century.
2. Midwives—Florida—Interviews. 3. Obstetrics—
Florida—History—20th century. I. Title.
RG961.F6S87   1988   618.2   87-5072
ISBN 0-8203-0950-8 (alk. paper)

British Library Cataloging in Publication Data available

Contents

	Preface	vii
	Note to Readers	xi
	Introduction	1
Chapter One	Charismatic Leader The Community's View of the Midwife	9
Chapter Two	Public Health Menace The State's View of the Midwife	34
Chapter Three	The Uneasy Meeting of Tradition and State	50
Chapter Four	A Rebirth of American Midwifery	69
	The Interviews	73
Appendix	A Long Dark Night The Midwives of Florida	223
	Notes	235
	Selected Bibliography	247
	Index	251

Preface

I remember an excited, Italian-American aunt pointing in reverent whispers at the very spot in her living room where my grandfather's coffin had rested. And if this was not enough to widen my young but urbane eyes, the tour continued upstairs with a run-through of the rooms in which she had "personally" given birth to her four children. My American predilection for modernism was sufficiently appalled! I had no acquaintance with a not-so-distant past in which the intervention of specialists was seldom available and even less desired. In the earlier parts of this century, in the Northern ethnic neighborhoods and the Southern rural towns, the resources one depended on were one's own—those and the resources of thirty-some-odd relatives (one of the advantages of extended-family life). And when these resources were exhausted and the roof was *still* leaking, there was always *somebody* you knew in the community who could fix it. Most needs could be met this way—intimately. And with such a coterie of talent, money often need not even change hands. Back in the old Italian neighborhood, where hand-stuffed sausage was adequate payment for the services of a midwife, it was common for women to attend one another at birth, common for nursing mothers to breastfeed each other's children, and so not at all unusual that I should have both a grandmother to the north and a grandmother to the south who each attended her share of childbirths. They did it out of necessity, out of a more intimate, shared experience, and in the context of a more separate female domain.[1] *Most* women took their turn at the birthing bed, sometimes in it and sometimes alongside it. Still, set apart from the dabbling female relatives and neighbor ladies, there was a smaller group of special women, particularly in the black South, who were recognized by the community as "midwives."

The American midwife's misfortune was to lose not only her vocation but her history as well. Segments of the medical community and state health bureaucracies appointed themselves the guardians of both, thus usurping the recognition and respect the midwife had earned from her community. Currently there are only two major works on the history of American midwifery,[2] and detailed information on the history of midwifery in Florida is scant when it appears at all. Jule Graves was a state health nurse directly involved with the development of the midwife program in Florida. Records from her estate have recently been added to the Florida State Archives in Tallahassee. These include not only numerous photographs, records, and correspondence, but a miniature replica of the birthing mannequin she designed and sought to patent. Florida's history is rich. There remains a handful of traditional midwives still practicing in some rural counties; current legislation on the issue has been revived (1983); and Florida's midwives represent three distinct cultures: the black, native American, and Latin communities.

Information in this study has come mainly from the black midwives of Florida, though the original intent was to span ethnic and geographical demarcations. However, after listening to the descendants of some Northern ethnic midwives, I realized that any detailed work on midwives from specific regions and backgrounds would need to reflect these differences and treat them separately. Though she may have been seen by her attackers as one entity to be rid of, the midwife's cultural situation was the context for her role in the community, and that naturally affected the expressions of her trade—that is, lore, remedies, training, and so on. The unifying factor was community regard; the seasoned midwife held a place of respect within her own community. But one would never know that from extant materials. While there are doctors and bureaucrats who have prolifically addressed the "midwife problem," little information has come from the midwife herself or her descendants or the community she served. These voices will prevail in the first chapter, as its title indicates. They turn up again in the interviews, transcribed with as little editing as possible. I debated the style the interviews would take—should I print them in "proper" English, or should I attempt to duplicate the sounds of accents and idioms that delighted my own (subjective) ear? The personalities of these women were as seductive as their stories, and I have tried to reflect this in the transcriptions. But I am still not certain that the way I have presented their words would not offend them. They are amiable oral historians. And the full appreciation of oral history requires the senses of sight and sound. To remedy this, I have produced a half-hour videotape of four of these interviews presented in documentary style. The written word alone does not do them justice.

Note to Readers

Because of the current controversial nature of this subject in Florida, all names of midwives and friends have been changed. The names of doctors, health officials, and Florida municipalities are represented by their first letter only, when taken from the interviews. When these appear in public documents, the names are printed in full. All the interviews included here were done with traditional black midwives in Florida over a three-year period, 1981–1984.

Introduction

In this century's earliest years, the medical profession, in league with state health officials, found virtually no statistics on the number or kinds of midwives practicing in the United States. If they were to protect the public from what they considered to be the midwife health menace, it would be helpful to know first just how widespread that menace was. So in the 1930s, three organizations conducted independent studies to gather data on the high U.S. infant and maternal mortality rates.[1] With all the recent medical "advances," why did this country's maternal mortality rate *increase* from sixty-one deaths per ten thousand live births in 1915 to seventy deaths in 1929? Why was it that neonatal deaths accounted for half of all infant deaths under one year? The answers were unexpected and, certainly for some, embarrassing.

All three studies placed blame squarely on the shoulders of the physician and his operative interference with the use of forceps, anesthesia, and surgery; exposure to the hospital's environment of cross infection was a correlative factor. Also, less than half of the graduating obstetric students had attended a birth by the time of graduation. The 1930

White House Conference on Child Health and Protection found that 65 to 80 percent of the childbirths in the United States required operative intervention, while Scandinavian countries and England reported only 15 percent. The New York Academy of Medicine's Committee on Public Health Relations cited as "preventable" 66 percent of its city's 2,041 maternal deaths between 1930 and 1933. Of these, physicians were responsible for 61.1 percent, while those attributed to midwives' errors were 2.2 percent. Out of one thousand live births, maternal death rates were distributed as follows: with physicians in attendance, 5.4; with surgeons, 9.9; and with midwives, 1.4. Though surgeons handled the more difficult cases, in normal labors the midwives' success rates were more than adequate, especially considering that their clients, due to economic circumstances, were thought to be higher-risk mothers. All three studies produced statistics that were favorable to the midwife's practice, though her opportunities for training were judged to be poor. The third study, by the Committee on the Costs of Medical Care, disclosed that the "midwife is not the determining factor in the country's high maternal mortality rate"; in fact, "untrained midwives approach, and trained midwives surpass, the record of physicians *in normal deliveries.*" The other two studies produced similar conclusions. But then, in defiance of all logic, they all agreed that "it is both undesirable and unlikely that the midwife as she is generally known in the United States today should have a permanent place in medical care in this country." Each recommended that concentration for improvements should go to upgrading physicians within the field of obstetrics.

There were a few who argued for the training of midwives and keeping midwifery as a respectable alternative. Dr. J. H. Mason Knox of the Maryland State Bureau of Child Hygiene said that it was "a little presumptuous for even well-qualified obstetricians to condemn midwives in general when our experience the world over is that in those countries in which midwives play the largest part in obstetric practice there is the lowest maternal mortality."[2] Members of the Subcommittee on Education of Midwives at the Washington conference presented Europe's impressive midwife statistics, raising them as a standard after which educational programs for American midwives might be modeled. But modern medical practice was having none of it. And though finding the midwife's statistics favorable, they were not as inclined to find a place in American health care for the forty-seven-thousand-plus practicing midwives.[3]

The context for the midwife's growing unpopularity in the United States was industrialization. The new technology of mass production was quickly shrinking the importance of the individual craftsman. The emphasis now was on efficiency and saving time. The midwife was a craftswoman, and the time she took to perform her craft was unfashionably slow and long, as was the natural course of labor and delivery. The hospital, on the other hand, employed technology to speed up and make "painless" the birth process; it was modeled after the modern factory—efficient, assembly-line care within a rigid schedule. The automated factory model, unlike its agrarian predecessor, required fewer laborers to accomplish its tasks. Large families were no longer the economic asset they once were, and the birthrate dropped accordingly, making childbirth an increasingly less common event, thus receiving more attention. The time was ripe for converting the previously ignoble field of obstetrics into a respectable, complex medical specialty. The nineteenth century saw the development of several technical inventions to be used in childbirth, and with each the gap between midwife and physician grew wider.[4] In 1808 Dr. John Stearns first used ergot to induce labor. In the 1820s, the stethoscope was used to monitor the fetal heartbeat through the mother's abdomen. With the use of anesthesia in surgery in the 1840s, Dr. Walter Channing encouraged the use of ether in normal as well as difficult births. Also in the 1840s, Oliver Wendell Holmes and Ignaz Semmelweis independently developed theories on the contagious nature of childbed fever (although this discovery was not generally applied in childbirth till later).

In the mid-1800s, J. Marion Sims designed a curved vaginal speculum, and in the 1870s, silver nitrate for the newborn's eyes was first used. As American culture gravitated toward science and technology, the obstetrician's practice appeared increasingly attractive by modern standards. Medical associations began recognizing obstetrics and gynecology as medical specialties, and once the barriers of modesty were broken, clinical demonstrations of live births became acceptable in teaching hospitals. Before the midwife ever became the physician's economic competitor, she was an obstacle to the refinement of his science. The midwife monopolized a large segment of the physician's prospective clientele; she was "taking up" the university hospital's "clinical material"—a rather cold designation for impoverished women who exchanged their pregnant bodies as classroom teaching models for free obstetrical care. Midwives were blamed for the physician's low status and economic rewards.

> Do you wonder that a young man will not adopt this field [obstetrics] as his special work? If a delivery requires so little brains and skill that a midwife can conduct it, there is not the place for him. . . . Parturition, viewed with modern eyes, is no longer a normal function, but that it has imposing pathologic dignity. . . . Only when the science of obstetrics were properly appreciated would the midwife be impossible to mention.[5]

Two inducements that lured a record number of women to their hospital beds were the pain-saving (or, more accurately, memory-depressing) Twilight Sleep and the time-saving forceps. The forceps were invented by Peter Chamberlen in the seventeenth century. After nearly a hundred years as the sole possession of the Chamberlen family, the forceps continued its status as an exclusive commodity—some physicians purchased the secret, while others invented their own. Finally the forceps became part and parcel of the physician-controlled hospital birth. Considering a *JAMA* article's admonition that motherhood should be "zealously guarded and cared for by trained physicians and not by ignorant midwives,"[6] it is not surprising that both the above innovations were monopolized by physicians, furthering the image of the midwife as a backward, old-world product. Still unimpressed, the midwife's last two American strongholds—the black women of the South and the immigrant women of the North—were tenacious in their loyalty to her. The low economic and educational status of these groups was conveniently used by physicians to further confirm hospital birth as the higher way. The racial and ethnic makeup of the women was used to play upon the "white" population's prejudices, remaking the midwife into some kind of un-American apparition and casting a suspicious shadow over her character as well as her work. A well-circulated ad depicted three midwives: an Italian woman, a Southern black woman, and an Irish woman, each dressed in dark, old-world garb and framed against an even darker background—a clear contrast to the slim, fashionable women of the adjoining ads. The ad's caption underscored the visual message:

A typical Italian midwife practicing in one of our cities. They bring with them filthy customs and practices. . . . A "granny" of the far South. Ignorant and superstitious, a survival of the "magic doctors" of the West Coast of Africa. . . . Surely, it might have been this woman of Irish-American parentage who is quoted as having said: "I am too old to clean, too weak to wash, too blind to sew; but, thank God, I can still put my neighbors to bed."[7]

Where modernity was not persuasive, the medical professionals found it necessary to launch a media campaign that would simultaneously discredit the midwife while promoting the relatively new idea (early nineteenth century) of pregnancy as pathological—a malady now requiring the highly trained physician and his technological bag of tricks. Popular women's magazines like *Good Housekeeping, Harper's,* and *Ladies' Home Journal*[8] bought the package and perpetuated this image in articles about the midwife—both fiction and fact—

while highlighting testimonials that touted the wonders of Twilight Sleep ("The Commotion, Noise, Hustle and Responsibility of one's Home or the General Hospital are all obviated.")[9] The threefold image of the midwife as "ignorant, dirty, and superstitious" sticks in the American unconscious even now, owing to the effectiveness of this early campaign.

For centuries, midwives had demonstrated labor and delivery for what it was—in most cases, an uncomplicated and natural process that required patience, confidence, and endurance. In communities where this was a given, the justification of obstetrics as a complex medical specialty proved untenable. And the midwife's adherents in the North and the South were resistant to both hospital birth and male doctors. The immigrants' language barrier served as a sanctuary for their customs, prolonging the immigrant midwife's practice and abating the English-speaking male accoucheur's encroachments. And in the South, rural black populations had little if any access to white hospitals, placing their midwives in competition with no one and consequently delaying their complete elimination for some time (a few black midwives still practice in Florida). Few doctors were optimistic that the midwife's "clients" would voluntarily give her up; so it was through the bureaucratic process of regulation that they sought to phase her out—almost imperceptibly. This approach met with no ostensible opposition inasmuch as the women who were being "phased out" had no public access for their own defense. The language, race, and education of the remaining midwives and their clients obstructed public expression and recognition of their plight. These as well as regional and economic factors impeded any united front against what appeared to be a beneficent and certainly legal crusade. The regulation of midwifery, though pursued on a state-by-state basis, generally conformed to the three-phase plan of education, licensing, and elimination. The advisory boards, consulting committees, and other bureaucratic groups to whom the responsibility of regulating the midwives fell would be heavily weighted with physicians—an extraordinary arrangement considering the financial competition between the two. The only possible outcome of such a relationship was the midwife's elimination.

The dissolution of the immigrant midwifery tradition came first. The Europeans viewed birth as a natural, ordinary process that was the province of women. The "foreign-speaking," male American doctor was called in only as a last resort—the midwife being a more reassuring, familiar connection with "home." A Philadelphia doctor in 1917 blamed unrestricted immigration for the continuing "midwife problem," which the practice of midwifery had come to be called by its detractors. He described the immigrants as people "ignorant in every sense of the word, who do not speak English, who have but little money, but are prolific breeders, and who come here with definite and fixed ideas in favor of the midwife rather than the doctor."[10]

The introduction of immigration-restriction laws in 1921 and 1924 enhanced the physician's practice over the midwife's. There was no longer the periodic influx of old-world cousins who, by example if not by harangue, reaffirmed European customs and language in the neighborhoods and homes of their new-world relations. And as each generation came of age, the desire to be Americanized was less clouded by ethnic tradition and loyalties. Of course, the midwife was one of these traditions, and hospital birth was the American way. And to be a true American woman, one was fashionably delicate in constitution, thus requiring whatever medical wonders could get her through this whole sordid childbirth ordeal. According to ethnic stereotypes, immigrant women (as well as black women in the South), on the other hand, had babies as easily as a cat had kittens—a sure indication of a cruder, more animal-like character.[11] These American-dream aspirations, coupled with the decreasing birthrate of the twenties and thirties, gradually put the Northern ethnic midwife out of business. By 1930, 80 percent of all midwives in the United States were located in the South.[12]

While the Northern midwife's demise was swift and final, the Southern midwife's elimination was strategic, prolonged, and more complex. State health officials viewed her as a necessary evil to be borne until medical services were improved. In the meantime, analogous but independent programs for the midwife's improvement were begun throughout the South under the jurisdiction of each state's board of public health. State health workers viewed themselves as rescuers of the public, especially the impoverished blacks, from antiquated birthing customs. Though generally sincere and respectful of the granny midwives, many state health workers regarded them as unfortunate women who were "pressed into service because there was no one else to deliver the babies." It was a "dismal picture" to be redressed by public health agencies, which had more direct contact with the midwives than did their more unkind critics, the physicians.[13] On the face of it, the aim of these programs was to educate and license the midwives, but the long-term plan was to replace the midwife with modern medical and hospital services, "to improve, regulate and—eventually—to eliminate midwifery."[14]

This would be a long time in coming. Hospital facilities often failed to reach outlying rural areas where black populations were densest, and under these circumstances Southern doctors had worked cooperatively with midwives as a necessity. What hospitals there were in the South were usually segregated, providing care to blacks only for emergencies and, even then, only in hospital-basement arrangements. But it was this segregated environment that bought the midwives some time.

Chapter One

Charismatic Leader

The Community's View of the Midwife

Beginnings

Down to the day we buried her, we received calls from everywhere.
People came from everywhere. And the one thing they wanted to talk
about was her work as a midwife, about what a good job she had
done. . . . A lady . . . had carried her son to the funeral home. . . . He
was about twenty-some years old . . . and he wanted to see this person
who had brought him into the world. . . . People thought there was
nothing like her. . . . [She] was a God-sent love to the whole community—black and white. . . . And some of 'em referred to her as Mother
Reynolds.[1]

Though most of the old midwives are dead now, still scattered
around this country are "her children," some, by now, carrying her
name to their own graves.[2] Her hands—poised and ready to "catch"
them—had given their skin its first human touch; her hands had ca-
ressed strength into their mothers' bodies; and her voice had been the
one low, even tone amidst those first sounds of wonder. She had many
children for a woman of her years, and that is why they called her

granny.[3] "They call it midwife. .... In them days, there was women—wasn't no doctor."[4]

There were two ways one assumed the title of midwife, and neither was voluntary. Many midwives were kin to, if not descendants of, other midwives—a reflection of an earlier time of family trades. Through an informal and, many times, unintentional apprenticeship, a daughter, granddaughter, or other female relative would occasionally go along to help the midwife on a birth. This style of on-the-job training, coupled with an unavoidable family involvement with the midwife's work, provided the younger woman with an evolving knowledge of childbirth and delivery—enough knowledge and experience that when the inevitable day arrived that the laboring woman was there and the midwife was not, it would fall to her, the unwilling apprentice, to "catch" the baby, solo.[5] It is not likely, at a time like this, that the word *no* would be offered or, what's more, accepted. For Evelyn, the daughter of a black urban midwife, that day came when she was thirteen years old.

This particular time, she had gone to check on a lady, and this lady, she came in—her husband brought her in like about eleven o'clock in the morning. I was at home, and this woman was rarin' to go. And I says, "Well, my God, Momma's not here." I didn't panic. I had seen her do it *so* many times. I just went right on in and got that paper tray and had him to put her little buttocks on that tray, scrubbed my hands, scrubbed her up and everything—I did this! I had seen my momma do it so many times. We were raised around this. So the baby just [slaps hands together] bob, just like that, here she comes, the little girl. After the baby was born, well, I knew better than to try to cut the umbilical cord, although I knew how to do it just as good. I'd seen my mother take the sterilized tape, tie it off, cut it, and how many inches to do it from the navel, but I wouldn't take a chance on *this*. I wrapped the baby up, made it very comfortable, 'cause she came here yellin'; there was no slappin' on the back. She just came here like, "Well, God, I'm glad to be here." The mother was very thrilled to see her here because evidently she'd been in a lot of pain, and the husband didn't think nothing of it. Then the baby started cryin'. "Well, you little rascal you," I said. "Evidently you want to eat." And I knew what my mother's philosophy was on that: always sterile sugar-water—sterilized bottle, nipple, water, and everything. I gave her about an ounce of sterilized water, and she drank. As my mother came, she was laying down in between her mother's legs just as comfortable and sound asleep. . . . My mother always instilled in us to be adults even when we were just children. And thank God that particular time she had because the husband probably would have just been frantic. But, I guess he could look at me and say, "Here's a thirteen year old just movin' just like the mother would have done." Yeah, yeah [laughter], he wasn't concerned at all; if so, he didn't say anything. And when my mother came, she said, "Look what we have here. Look what Evelyn did for us!" Of course, that child was named after me, and I'm real proud. I don't know where she is today, but she was named Evelyn after me.[6]

Once the novice successfully completed her first delivery, the push for her to take up the craft moved to a new level, and whether she liked it or not, proofs of her worthiness became the subject of community speculation. "The candidate" had now concretely demonstrated her aptitude for midwifery, and the old, sagacious midwives would henceforth regard her as the possessor of an inherited talent. She had exhibited a hereditary predisposition for midwifery that had been passed down from her older midwife relation(s). Most midwives had a strong desire to pass down their craft, especially to a member of the family. This ambition to keep the trade in the family was potent enough to move the Jacksonville bureaucracy.[7] Upon the death of her aunt, a longtime midwife, Mary Lee Jones sent a letter to the State Board of Health requesting permission to take up her aunt's practice—a request the office denied because "they had enough midwives." Mrs. Jones wrote back to let them know she *would* be practicing, inasmuch as her precursor had handed over her equipment to her with that intent. The license came to Mrs. Jones in the return mail. In addition to her aunt,

Mrs. Jones's mother and grandmother were midwives. It was the same with other midwives in the black community; one woman claimed a grandmother, a mother, and a mother-in-law—all midwives.

Midwifery was not a science; it worked respectfully *with* nature (midwife translates "with-woman"). Unlike obstetrics (which translates "to stand in the way"), midwifery was noninterventive. Since the mother's body naturally performed the task of delivering a child, the hallmark of a good midwife had more to do with personal qualities than technical skills (though certainly competence was enhanced with time). Should these charismatic attributes become manifest to a veteran midwife adept at spotting them, woe to the unwilling apprentice!

> Well, a lady lived down the street there. She was a midwife, and she'd gotten old. She said, "I'm gettin' old; somebody got to take it." I'd been with her several times, and she just kept on asking me about joinin' the board, but I didn't *want* to be a midwife. So I kept pushin' her off until at last, one day, my grandson was born here. My daughter had her baby okay; she sits back and lets me deliver the baby. I did the cord and everything and dressed the baby. The old midwife looked at me and laughed. She said, "Why don't you come on and go to the meetin' Friday?" I said, "I will." I'd be gettin' her off my back, you know. She kept so closely; I said, "Well, I'm goin'." So really that Friday I went, and after I joined the board, then everywhere she went, every time she got a call, she would call me 'cause I was drivin' a car. And she would go on and call me and tell me to come where she was. And I did that. In a year's time, I had got my license.[8]

Much to the chagrin of the old midwives, there were some women who were as stubborn as they were talented, and it took a little more than a few accidental deliveries, community pressure, and midwife relations to convert them to their "calling." After all, who could better attest to the erratic hours and weighted responsibilities of the midwife than a midwife's daughter? For Johnnie Seeley, being the granddaughter of a midwife was more a hindrance than an incentive for her joining "the board" in her midthirties.⁹ Only the most dramatic appeals could crack the resistance of some; and more often than not, a provocative occurrence was the last and most effective argument to convince the most obstinate to take on the mantle of midwife. Whether through visions or voices, prayers or dreams, few midwives—ordinarily religious women—could resist what clearly presented itself as a personal calling, whether directly from God or indirectly through a revered elderly midwife. And unless one was wont to repeat the mistake of Jonah and suffer his most unfortunate fate, there was only one response to a calling: you accepted it. As one Arkansas midwife put it, "If the Lord has something he wants you to do, you won't have no good luck unless you do it."¹⁰ What follows is a sampling of such occurrences:

> It was eighteen years ago, the eleventh of November. I had quilted out a quilt that day, all by myself. I finished it late at night and put it in the closet, said to myself, "Now, tomorrow morning I can begin another task." I sat down in front of the fire. Was tired, so tired. I sat there for awhile and rested, and then when I leaned over and started to untie my shoe, the spirit spoke to me. The spirit said, "You'll have to put those shoes back on before day." You understand that the spirit don't talk out loud like I'm talking now, but speaks low, like a deep reasoning in the heart.
>
> I stopped and folded my hands and looked in the fire, and went over the community in my mind to see if anybody was sick. But I didn't find nobody sick. Then I took off my shoes and bowed on my knees, laid my hands out in the chair I was sitting in, and prayed, "Lord, whatsoever my hands find to do, let me do it joyfully, and bless the work of my hands, and bless everything my hands have laid to for good. Lord, my eyes are dim, strengthen my eyes so I can see; my knees are weak, strengthen my knees so I can run on your erruns." Then I got up and went to bed, and right off to sleep.
>
> Way in the night, Jake—who lives a mile down the road—called at my winder, "Mis' Ada, get up. I want you to go down home." Through my sleep, I asked him what was the matter. He said Inez was sick, and he

wanted me to come and wait on her. So I got up and sponged my body
with cold water, like I do every morning, put on my shoes, rushed out of
the door, and run all the way to Jake's house.

When I got there, the baby was ready born. I didn't have no medicine bag
then like I got now, and I never had cut a cord. So I knelt down on the
floor by the mother and baby and kept asayin', "Lord, now help me do
this right. Show me how, Lord, show me how." Then I tied and cut the
cord, and it didn't bleed a speck. I got the mother and baby up on the bed
and scoured the floor. . . . All tired out, I went to the kitchen and pushed
out the shutter. And there it was a beautiful morning, the sun was rose just
above the trees. Then it all came back to me what the spirit had spoke.
Before the daylight, I had put on my shoes, I had run, and I had done all
that work, and now the sun was just a-coming up. Hadn't I asked the Lord
to strengthen my knees? Hadn't I asked Him to bless the work of my
hands?

From that day, I've borned seventy-five babies, white and colored, and I
ain't lost a one in birth, mother or baby.[11]

In the case of Mary Beth Chambers, the Lord spoke not to Mrs.
Chambers, but, as she tells it, to her mentor, Eliza Overton:

It was a lady named Eliza Overton. She's dead. That's the one I trained
under. She delivered a baby in J——. She said she was wantin' to quit, and
she had went to Dr. S—— and told him that she was gonna stop. She was
old, and she was tired. He say, "Well, you got to get somebody." And she
went to studyin' and prayin' and say I come before her one night. She had
delivered a baby right in this community, down in the mine corp—when
the mine was all abloom. And she come back to check the baby like we
always do. When she come back, she sent for me to come down to the
house where she was at. And when I went, she said, "Now, you who I
wanta see." She said, "Friday, I want you to meet me in H—— and go to
Q—— with me. I want to turn you in to the clinic. I want you to take my
place." And I said, "Well, Eliza, I don't particularly want to be no midwife. I've been with the doctor at home. A white lady I used to work with,
I was with the doctor with her. With all of hers, I was the midwife, but I

just assist him." She had hers at home, you know, and I'd be there with her. I say, "I don't wanta deliver no babies." She said, "Yeah, I want you to. I'm comin' on. Dr. S—— said I had to get somebody in my place. I pray to the Lord, and I saw you. You stood right before me, and I want you to take my place." She was a sweet old lady. I wouldn't deny her. I got up that mornin', got my husband to take me to H——. We caught the bus. When I got there, she was there. And we went on to Q—— to the clinic. So she turned me in and told the nurses she was gonna be with me until I make my rounds and get my license. And she did.[12]

Not all midwives approached the birthing bed with such reluctance. For some, it was an idea they had nurtured for a long time. Both Rosalind Stephenson and Georgia Reynolds were said to have passed up the traditional child's game of "doctor" for a more interesting invention called "midwife." They took turns delivering the "babies" of sisters, friends, and unsuspecting pets. Though called by God, Mrs. Jones's inspiration originated in childhood, too. With three midwives in the family, as a child Mary Lee was regularly evicted from her home when a birth was in progress. On one occasion, feeling determined, she crawled under the house and lay quietly to hear the first cries of a baby born in the room above her. From that moment on, it was her obsession. Mrs. Stephenson was equally undaunted. After years of watching the work of her grandmother and aunt, Mrs. Stephenson developed such a love for the craft that she "snuck in" on the births of the county's best midwife in a sort of clandestine apprenticeship. Later a cousin asked her to help deliver her baby. The older midwife inspected Mrs. Stephenson's handiwork and deemed it worthy but would not show her how to fill out the birth certificate, fearing the competition this new upstart might bring to her own practice. Mrs. Stephenson found her way around that and willingly began her thirty-five-year practice. She came to love it, as did even the most unwilling beginners.

Whether she came by it pragmatically or with a touch of high drama, the midwife's beginnings launched a lifetime vocation—one that would make her a respected leader among both men and women of her community. And more than her delivery skills, her personal qualities—patience, empathy, a kind of innate wisdom—gave her leadership its charismatic flavor. Unlike members of the ordinary medical profession, the midwife did not "pick" her profession but was chosen by it—sometimes divinely. Mrs. Jones attributed her skills to God, who gave them to her through her long line of midwife relations. The midwife did not *acquire* her talents but already had them: they comprised the basis for her calling. One midwife said she was born a granny: "God made me dat way."[13] Another related the spiritual dimensions of midwifery:

> The good Lord taught me how to catch babies. . . . I don't know how many babies I caught; must have been more than 1,000, both black and white babies. . . . When I was catching babies, I would pray for you. I would ask the Lord to help you and to help me to take care of you. I've prayed so hard, and my soul would be so full of joy. . . . I never used any instruments.[14]

Birth Among Women

> They'd have women in t'hold their hand, or heat water'r'somethin'. There was always somethin' to do. They always had four, five women plus a doctor [midwife].[15]

The birthing chamber was the focal point of a variety of deep female attachments: there was the relationship between the laboring woman and her midwife; the midwife and former "clients"; the laboring woman and her mother, grandmother, sister, or other supporting female relative(s); and the laboring woman and her friends. All were there to assist her through this experience that, were this her first baby, would induct her into the sorority of women who had given birth. It was an intimate occasion, a lengthy ordeal, and one that, like little else in their lives, was controlled exclusively by the women. Let there be a hint of an impending birth, and the women would gather together, asked or not, to work toward the common goal of helping another woman at "her time." It was both an event of consequence and a felicitous social occasion. Our colonial foremothers attached the custom of "groaning parties" to their childbirths. Once mother and baby were settled and well, the appreciative mother would throw a banquet for the women who were present at her birth. The name was reminiscent of the groans of labor as well as the groans of the women who would undoubtedly stuff themselves at the feast.

The attachment women felt for their midwives is reflected in those who took what often was their last birth to the hospital when their midwife died. A hospital birth was preferable to replacing a long-standing midwife. The connection between mother and midwife was more than functional—it was personal (particularly for women whose *mothers* were their midwives). After looking on the familiar and reassuring face of the midwife present at all previous births, to have anyone else attending seemed nothing less than an intrusion.

Mrs. Wilson, herself a midwife, chose to give birth alone when her mother and sister—both midwives—were unavailable. She would call no one else, but instead delivered her own baby on her knees. She said that just to have her mother in the same room with her could chase a headache away. This kind of confidence was echoed in the memories women shared about their midwives. One could not come away from their wistful descriptions without realizing the intensity of respect and fondness the midwife had evoked in them. When Jenny Black's midwife died at ninety, there was nowhere else to take her last birth but to the hospital. After all, it was this same midwife who had attended her mother when she (Mrs. Black) was born—a midwife whose work spanned two generations. The relationship had been too personal to even consider having another; and the hospital was the more unsentimental choice. What woman could follow an act like that?

By the time I got in the hospital, I had broke my water. I told them to call the doctor; they didn't. They says it wasn't time. She say, "Who the nurse?" I say, "You, but I'm the one deliverin' the baby." She *still* wouldn't call the doctor. . . . And you know, she picked up a towel, a big ol' bath towel, and rolled that thing and balled it up. She put it down here [points to her vagina] and got another one and crossed my legs. And I said, "Uh-uh, oh, no, you won't kill me like *this!*" [She was trying to] keep the baby from coming, and the child was so near. The doctor wasn't there, you know, and then I was in the bed [not the delivery room]. Oh, she was going on, "Blow out ja' mouth, blow out ja' mouth." The pain struck me so hard. I took my foot and shoved her over to that wall. [Laughter.] I wasn't gonna let her kill me and the child. By the time they got me in the delivery room and throwed me over there, that child's *head* came. And by the time he [the doctor] walked in, the child was almost all the way here. [The nurse] didn't even prep me. See, she waited so late, then she was goin' to prep me. I said, "Well, you ain't goin' to put no razor on me." And, whoa, them pains hit me, and I'm jumpin'. "You just have to be still." I said, "Nuh-uh, . . . you ain't gonna put that razor on me, and I mean it." I had a little ol' jar of deodorant that I got, and I was gonna let her have it. 'Cause I won't let her cut me with that razor. Because she didn't have any right. I kept telling her that it was time. . . . Then she say, "You have a baby like a cat have kittens." I go, "Well, you must be the cat had the kittens."[16]

The Florida State Board of Health records show that in 1943 Alberta Hinson succeeded her mother, Sallie Dixon, who retired. Most of the families who once called on Sallie Dixon would now call on Alberta Hinson. Since the midwife's daughter, in her apprenticeship—whether formal or informal—had accompanied her mother on previous rounds, many families were already familiar with the "new" midwife, and the transition was a smooth one. It was as if a part of the old midwife still remained. Continuity of family lines was maintained at both ends of the birthing bed. When the number of years between generations was small, a woman in labor might be attended by the same midwife who delivered her from *her* mother; or she and her mother, being pregnant at the same time, might share the same midwife. This tight family network of women was the last stronghold that, for years, most effectively warded off the medical profession's incursions into the birthing room. Childbirth was directed by women over many generations; it was a woman's ritual.

During labor, the midwife's tasks were as varied as her imagination. In the first stages of labor, her immediate concern was to make the mother as comfortable as possible, both physically and mentally. Some midwives brought along their Old Testaments, from which they would read encouraging passages, the Psalms being a common favorite. Other midwives, like Augusta Wilson, avoided this when attending younger first-time mothers, concerned that the woman might associate these readings with death and become afraid. Mrs. Wilson preferred to get their minds off the pain: "[I] joke around and cut the fool with 'em and tease 'em and go on. And after awhile, they get to laughing and talking and relax theyselves. And sometimes, first thing, here the baby, and then some don't think about the pains or what they was going through."[17] As to practical matters, the midwife might bring chewing gum or hard candy for the mother to suck on; she would fan her, put cool pads on her face, massage hands, hips, and whatever parts of her laboring body needed attention. And she talked with her—sometimes all night—allowing her to walk around during early labor. For long labors the midwife might have a cot or bed on which she could lie down close to the mother, if she were attending the woman alone. When assistants were at hand, she took brief trips back to her own home, leaving other women to watch the mother's progress (but only during early labor). There was usually enough for everyone to do, but when there were more women than tasks, most midwives preferred a crowd of fewer numbers. When the crowd began to interfere with the mother's concentration, it was time for the midwife to exercise her authority.

If a midwife did not exercise this control, the outcome was potentially tragic, as was the experience of Mrs. Wilson. While attending the birth of a young first-time mother, the woman's relatives, who were of the Holiness faith, were in attendance, rocking to and fro with religious fervor. With the onset of labor's final stages, the women's behavior grew more frenetic—"jumpin' and shoutin' and . . . 'thank God and holy come on Jesus!' "[18] At this, the woman became so afraid and nervous that her contractions stopped altogether. Recognizing the danger, Mrs. Wilson insisted her patient be taken to the hospital. And only after much wrangling with the relatives (*they* had never had to go to the hospital!) did they rush her to the emergency room, only in time to see the baby die. Mrs. Wilson, without benefit of a hearing, had her license revoked (see pp. 48–49).

With mother and baby's safety as her first priority, the midwife needed to be firm when the situation called for it: "So I say, 'Now if you got a friend, she can come in and help ya.' But all this other crew runnin' in to see a baby born, they gettin' out. Wait till they have theirs, and then they'll see it. I don't care. They know me—I won't play it."[19]

It was more common that the judgment of the midwife was heeded. In fact, many women believed the midwife "knew" when the baby would come: "She know the hour." Whether from years of experience or from an intuition born of her charismatic role, the midwife was thought by some to have an inside track on such things. But for the occasional skeptic, persuasion was usually meted out with patience and humor; for the midwife persona was nothing else if not imposing.

One girl, me and her grandmother was waitin' on her, and the girl went in her room and locked the door. [Laughter.] When she locked the door, she had a pain. "Ah! Mis' Rosalind, come 'ere, come 'ere." I say, "Uh-uh! You done locked me out. I ain't comin', I ain't comin'." "Mis' Rosalind, won't you get in my room!" I say, "I ain't comin' *nowhere!*" Ooooooh! When that pain was up, I bet she didn't lock that door no more. [Laughter.] Oh, I have so much fun with 'em.20

The midwife relied on the fact that a young mother unaccustomed to the intensity of labor would eventually come around to the midwife's "point of view"—labor pains provided a powerful argument.

I had one girl I delivered, she wouldn't stay in the bed. She wouldn't do nothin'. She just climbed and twist. I could never work with her; I went right along with her. She say, "Well, alright, I'm gonna go out the door." And I said, "Well, go ahead on; you'll come back." I didn't go out; I didn't follow her. She went out on the back porch. I stayed right there by that bed. And when the right pain hit her, she came back. [Laughter.] I've had 'em fightin', bitin', do everythin'.21

The midwife's services did not end with the safe delivery of the baby. Her last task was to direct a period of confinement for the mother—most commonly, nine to ten days. The midwife would prescribe bed rest with a cautious eye to diet—and each case called forth a different prescription. The women who remember observing this confinement confided that they believed ten to be an arbitrary if not excessive number, but it was a ritual they observed just the same. What then, if not health, was the reason behind 240 bedridden hours? It was during this time that the mother was visited by midwife, friends, and relatives, who saw to both her and her family's needs. One rural Southern woman said her midwife *stayed* at the house for two weeks after her birth, cleaning and watching her diet and generally caring for the baby and mother. Mrs. Wilson recalled using both pre- and postnatal times to teach young mothers how to sew. The length of time the midwife would linger after the birth depended on the needs of the mother. It was at least long enough to check the mother's recovery; and for first-time mothers, it was helpful to have someone around to offer pointers on caring for the new baby. In an informal survey of women who had their births at the hospital, those suffering from what "experts" call postpartum depression traced its source to a lack of emotional support from immediate others. They did not sense from husbands and friends a full appreciation for, and thus a sharing of, the intensity of responsibility they had just undertaken as mothers.[22] After the excitement died down and the mother-in-law flew home, the women reported feeling quite alone in their new avocation. The midwife and family model of confinement seems to have eased this adjustment. It was a ritual that answered emotional and practical needs.

When asked about the recent trend of inviting fathers into the birthing room, many midwives regarded the notion as amusing; and with rolled eyes or mild hysterics they would immediately launch into their favorite inept-husband story. But a couple of the *mothers* reacted more strongly, exhibiting nothing short of a fierce defense of their *right* to an all-female birth. Aside from a modesty indigenous to their time, many women looked upon childbirth as a direct blessing from God to woman: "What God gave me I want for myself!" Eve's curse of guilt and pain in childbirth was consistently rejected by women who otherwise put great store in the Bible. The negative elements associated with birth by the Judeo-Christian tradition were in direct conflict with the women's experiences. Not wanting to repudiate Scripture, but struggling to expound the passage, their interpretations ranged from mild distortions to out-and-out heresies. This positive approach to birth, nurtured in a women-directed setting, was coupled with a historical context in which women exercised this much direct and exclusive power over little else. What resulted was a sort of intangible women's club, a universal sisterhood of women who had been inducted into the rites of motherhood. Just the sight of a young pregnant woman could illicit nods of approval from the front-stoop matriarchs of the ethnic neighborhoods. One woman noticed that it was women, not men, who were more deferential to her in public when she was pregnant—giving up their seats or making way for her.[23]

Birth among women was an event of power, not the powerless ordeal of the hospital. And the distortion of its meaning by people who had not and would never give birth—i.e., men—was as great a factor as any for keeping them out. Mrs. Stephenson generally objected to the inclusion of husbands and boyfriends at her deliveries. She was concerned that a man would use some part of what he had witnessed at his woman's delivery as a point of embarrassment to her in later arguments.[24] He might turn her event of power into an object of ridicule. Male distortion of this female experience also came in the form of well-meaning misinterpretation. Midwife advocates often use the argument that, not having ever had a baby, the male doctor is subject to misread the nonverbal messages of his patient—a form of communication that, at some stages, may be all a laboring woman can or will articulate. Interpreting the pleading look in his patient's eyes as a cry for relief from pain, the doctor, feeling compelled to *do* something, responds with drugs—perhaps as much for his own relief as for hers. The midwife, recognizing the look as a need for emotional support, responds with her words, eyes, and touch to say that what is happening to you now has happened many times before; it is *supposed* to be like this; I personally know how you are feeling. The natural process of birth requires not intervention, but endurance; and the "expert" in this field is the one who has endured. In a survey of over two hundred mothers, including women who chose to have a hospital birth, informants rated their doctor's advice as last and friends' first as most useful to them. "When you get through going through seven months of examinations, and you share that special moment with him, I mean you just want to hug him. It would be nice to have a relationship with your doctor on a different level. I always wished that the doctor could share in this sort of spiritual celebration of birth."[25] The woman going through pregnancy, labor, and delivery with a midwife, however, did experience the relationship on a deeper level.

> I had 'em [babies] for midwives because midwives come to see you all the time. Now, she might miss this morning; she'll come and find out how you gettin' along before you have the baby. Yes, she stay there till it's all over with. . . . They'll sit down and talk to you how to do and not to eat. That's all was going with no doctors, 'cause they never come in them days. Nothin' but midwives. And they just cut off all those midwives. There no midwives to wait on nobody that I think about. Ain't never hear talk of none. But I believe they should go back and *get* those midwives.[26]

After birth, women shared the responsibility for one another's children. When need arose, *one* woman might breastfeed another's child. A few women from my group of informants had raised other people's children besides their own; sometimes these were so-called illegitimate children of relatives. Whether or not women-attended birth had anything to do with the ease of these arrangements, simply participating in the birth of a friend's child made one that much closer to that child's welfare.

At a time when few women could boast position or property, they were in the birthing room, outside the realm of men, bequeathing personal power and camaraderie to their daughters. The relatively recent absence of this women's tradition in the United States coincides with a more divisive connection between mothers and daughters in regard to birth. It was one Irish-immigrant midwife's custom to call in her two oldest granddaughters to help midwife their mother's births; the family circle was complete with three generations of women in attendance. Though many younger women that I interviewed opted for a midwife birth, few desired to have their mothers present at the delivery. Many believed that their mothers, if asked, would be equally resistant to the idea. Such resistance from both mothers and daughters is a product of the state's successful obliteration of a tradition—one that cultivated female solidarity and strength. These are different times than the days when a midwife's daughter would come 350 miles just to have her own mother deliver her baby, as did the daughter of a north-Florida midwife, Beckie MacBride. The connection of mother and daughter at the birth of a new family member transcended all disputes, all estrangements. Contemporary women's consciousness-raising and rap groups are perhaps a contrived and desperate attempt to revitalize this kind of intimacy among women, but they do not even approach the bond among women who have spent many hours alone together waiting up for a birth.

The Toil and Travail of Midwifery

Somewhere in the mountains I sit in the kitchen with Emma, an Appalachian midwife. Seated in her living room, rapidly depleting what seems like a carton of cigarettes, are two women, a mother and daughter. We can hear them talking as they wait, but they are not waiting to see Emma; they are waiting for the young woman's baby to be born. But *that* is not due to happen for another two weeks, and yet the daughter appears to have moved in for the duration. On another visit to Emma's home two or three years prior, a friend reported noticing three to four of these opulently figured women, all waiting, dispersed amongst the living-room furniture—the room being dominated by an old four-poster bed. Emma, with cheerful aplomb, tends to her daily routine of raising a garden and goats and chickens until the time nears for a delivery. She credits her automatic washer and drier for the ease with which, at eighty-four, she manages these myriad chores. Meanwhile, a large older woman comes in. She takes what is apparently her accustomed chair in the next room and just sits, joining in the waiting and conversation still in progress.

Emma tells me the old woman comes to her for doctoring. Through a series of interruptions that include the oft-ringing telephone, a visit from a granddaughter, and the one-liners an old farmer and buddy of Emma's husband is relating loudly for the benefit of my tape recorder, we complete the interview. Her pride is showing as she leads me to the birthing room located at the house's farthest (and quietest) end, on the other side of the kitchen. Inside its door, the cool tones of blue and white pacify this light space; filmy white curtains blow toward us, and two single, white, chenille-spreaded beds face each other on opposing blue walls. And there is an old incubator here—the one the county health department gave to Emma when they acquired their own newer model. On the wall is a photo taken on the day it was donated. The officials are wearing their faces of respect—something state bureaucrats rarely donned for midwives. But then, how many of these "officials" go *way back* with Emma?

Emma is prototypical both of the array of services a midwife provided for her community and of the veneration they mirrored back. For the midwife who made home deliveries—and most of them did—there was much more to be done than catching a baby, and plenty of waiting time in which to do it. If there were no relatives or neighbors to which the mother's custodial chores could be assigned, the midwife did them. Labor did not alter the need for children to be fed, bathed, and tucked in; and a woman's labor was not helped if she worried over tasks left undone. When poverty was a factor, the midwife would show the mother how to prepare hand-sewn sanitary pieces. In addition to the sanitary napkins she would need after birth, they would prepare a large birthing pad upon which she would deliver. All would be sterilized in the oven, wrapped, and stored. The midwife's usual high standard of cleanliness was not always satisfied by some of the homes she visited; for these she brought along sterile linen from home. At Mrs. Reynold's maternity home, the bed sheets were individually starched and ironed by the midwife herself. And for the more repulsive conditions, a midwife could require a change of venue. Mrs. Stephenson once ordered a family to exterminate the roaches in their home before she would deliver a baby there. Working in other people's homes required that a midwife be flexible and inventive.

When a woman became a midwife, it was a responsibility that would affect her entire family—especially if the children were still at home. If nothing else, the unpredictable hours were disruptive to any semblance of family continuity. The hardship of travel was often a shared chore; husbands, sons, and daughters took turns accompanying the midwife on night calls or in bad weather.

> Somebody's in labor, and it's pouring down rain, oh, my Lord. I know I went to Georgia one night, and my husband in there, before he died, he said, "Well, you shore is crazy. I [bet ya before I'd get out from here], they'd take that woman and carry her on to the hospital or somewhere." But I went, and I've did that several times now. Talk about praying—but pray then because an old piece of car, it's dark on the road, you don't know when you're gonna run in the ditch or somethin' gonna run into ya. And you had to carry the Lord wit'cha. But I always had good success, good luck. I never had no problems.[27]

Sometimes a midwife would attend two births simultaneously—driving between two points, maybe two counties, or crossing the state line. Perhaps all she would see of her home for two days was the outside of it as she drove by on her way to a birth. Some busy urban midwives resolved this home-and-work conflict by opening maternity facilities near their homes. This was the resolve of three women in my sample. Georgia Reynolds's initiative and ingenuity are representative:

> I must have been about fifteen or sixteen years old at the time when it opened because we were young teenagers, and [my mother] didn't want us to be home alone. That was her reason for setting up the clinic at home. She didn't want to be away from home. She wanted to be able to peep in on the family as well as to do her work. . . . About the late forties and

early fifties is when she built that home. And building that home, she started a career for another member of her family. She told my uncle, "I gotta have a building." She says, "I know just how I want it built." And he says, "What do you mean you're goin' to have a building?" "Well, I'm going to bring my work home." And my father said, "Well, you must be crazy. You're out of your mind talkin' about building a maternity home." [Laughter.] And she just got out there, and she figured out how long a bed was and how wide a bed was and how many feet and inches it would take up. She knew how many she wanted to have on each side of the wall. She must have had about a ten- or twelve-feet span. She wanted it large enough to be able to wheel 'em from the delivery room into their bed area. And it was an open ward type thing with windows on each side, and eventually she put an air conditioning system in and everything. And my uncle, who was also a person who did *not* finish school, but was a person who was always very skillful, had never laid any block in his life. She said, "But you can do it. I'm going to show you how to do it." Now, she had never laid any either. So he ended up building that place at the corner of B—— and 22nd on a very busy street in T——. And *so* many people passed; they saw his work, they liked his work. He didn't know what he was doin', but he started a career that lasted another thirty-some years in the building trade. Mm-hmm.[28]

Bringing the practice home further increased the family's involvement and turned the midwife's practice into a kind of family business. Evelyn kept the books for her mother and helped out during her teenage years—even on days, she confessed, when she would have much preferred to be at majorette practice. Her brother was finally relieved of his responsibilities when a woman he was transporting to the maternity home nearly delivered herself of her child in his car. Being sixteen, male, and sufficiently frightened—not to mention embarrassed—he swore never to make another pickup for his mother, who, appreciating his point, never asked him again.

It is a good thing that most midwives were steadfastly in love with attending childbirth, because payment for services had always been shaky at best. With doctors making an average of nearly five to ten times the cost of a midwife (Mrs. Stephenson quoted her charge at $125; the doctors of her area charged $1,200), most midwives also expressed a concern for the poor: "I just felt like there's *somebody* got to do somethin'. I'm gonna die one day, and I can be a help to somebody. And so out of my auntie dying, my grandma dying . . . this what worry me now: they cut out all the midwives, who is goin' to help these poor peoples what not able? That's the way I feel about it."[29] And so, few who came to the midwife could expect to be turned away. The work of attending women in childbirth and helping them deliver their babies is truly a work of the heart. "I went if I had t' crawl," is how one midwife expressed her commitment.

Many of the midwives repeatedly spoke of their love for their vocation and a corresponding sadness at no longer being able to practice. When phased out, few had yet attained their commonly held desire to deliver triplets. Most had delivered a few sets of twins, but triplets!—now there was something to look forward to. On the day I went to see Emma in Tennessee, she had just lost a chance to attend a woman who was expected to have multiple births. The woman's mother, at the last minute, backed out of their arrangement and took her daughter to the hospital, saying that her daughter was "allergic" to pain. The disappointment in Emma's voice was clear when she said, "I do hopes I lives to deliver triplets." Emma is eighty-seven.

Since midwives love babies, the more babies the better. Reportedly, the exhilaration one feels from the delivery of a multiple birth is enough to rob you of a night's sleep—that is, unless you deliver *two* sets in one day, as Mrs. Jones did: "That day I was too tired. I couldn't do nothin' *but* go to sleep." One midwife in my sample did deliver the much-coveted triplet birth, and she told me the story:

> The girl didn't have no hot water. The mother went over there and come back with a pan of hot water. So when she come, I say, "Now, Pam, this stupid gal got *two* babies!" She had the pan of water. "What you say,

Rosalind?" I say, "She got twins!" [Claps her hands.] Just dropped the
whole pan of water. [Laughter.] And I was so tickled, you know? "Bless
your soul." I say, "You get out from here and go get me some more water."
[Laughter.] She went and get some more water. When she come back, I
said, "*Pam*! Here *another* baby!" "Oh, goddamn!" [She acts out dropping
the pan again.] And honey, that woman, her momma tickled me so bad.
Them chillun, they go to school now. She had two boys and a girl.
[Laughter.] I can't help it—a crazy lady—just dropped *all* the water. I say,
"You better go ahead just get those sheets and wrap my babies up." And
they looked so pretty. So *I* wanted to have on my cap and my apron and
be there *with* the babies, but they went and had the babies' picture made
and put it in the papers.[30]

This love for babies transcended the social mores common to the
rest of the midwife's community. Not one midwife accepted the notion
of illegitimate children: "They's all children to me" was a commonly
shared sentiment. So when the topic of abortion came up, the answer
was easy: "No." Yet their conviction was not so much a moralistic
principle as an affirmation of all life as positive and legitimate, as they
knew it from their intimate familiarity with birth. A few midwives,
realizing the difficulties for some women in such a decision, were willing to cross yet another barrier—one of race—to lend support to those
choosing to go ahead with an unwanted birth. Their policy was to not
only deliver the child but to *raise* it, black or white, and then turn it
over to the mother if she, at some future date, decided she wanted it
back. One midwife tried to accommodate both the state and women
who wanted the father's name on the birth certificate. She would sometimes delay turning in a birth certificate for a few days if a woman was
going to marry the father within that time, thus allowing the midwife
to fill in his name at the last minute. The midwife traditionally placed
herself firmly in the camp of mothers and babies, where her highest
loyalties lay, rather than act as officiary of the state.

Lot of this abortion goin' on that shouldn't be. That ought to be lawed out—plum out. They'll be a lot of people suffer for that. They may not now, but they will later. They's been several called me about it. I told 'em I didn't do that. I said I wouldn't for the world. I said, "That's murder." They's a woman that come up here not too long ago. It's been about— well, she done had time to have it. Her and her sister both just sit here. Her sister sat over there, and they's both pregnant. Her sister said she wanted to come up here and have hers, and her husband wanted to go to the hospital—and, yes, she'd have to go to the hospital. This other 'un said she wanted me to do somethin' for her, help her do somethin'. I asked her what it was, and I told her if it was anything that wasn't honest and decent I wasn't gonna. She told her sister to tell me. So her sister said, "She wants you to help her have abortion." I said, "No, I don't do that." Now she said, "This baby don't belong to my husband, and I can't keep it. I've got to get rid of it." I just thought she oughtn't have stepped out on her husband if it didn't belong to him, but I didn't tell her that; I thought, though. I ought to, really. I told her, "That's murder." She said she'd been to the hospital; she'd been to see the doctors; and she'd been to the clinics; and there wasn't none of them. She's about twenty-two weeks 'cause she was showing then. They knowed that too far along, I guess. They just turned her down. I said, "Don't destroy that little baby, this life. If you want to," I said, "you carry on to its time if you will. Then you come up here, and I'll deliver it for you; or at least I'll do my best to deliver your baby." I said, "If you don't want it, then after you have it, just give it to me." I said, "You can get up and go home, and you won't even have to see it if you don't want to." She said, "I may have to do that; but if I get rid of it, I'm going to." She got up and left, and I never heard another word about 'em.[31]

The midwives were consistently women of strength and character, recounting a variety of accomplishments. A few had delivered their own babies without any assistance. Mrs. Jones had had such easy births and equal success at delivering others' babies that she saw no reason she shouldn't be able to deliver her own, and she did—three times. The respect the community held for the midwife is unmistakable. One midwife was recognized by her community for delivering a stillbirth; the baby weighed twenty pounds. She was asked to stand up before her church and was given a "diploma" by the local doctor, not to mention the write-up she received in a medical journal for her feat.

Midwives were invariably church women. Mrs. MacBride spoke proudly of her daughter the evangelist. Many believed firmly that they went on their rounds in the company and with the blessing of God. One rural midwife gave up her practice to pursue the responsibilities of a church for which she is both founder and minister. One night while closing up a rural grocery store, the Reverend Eva Brown said she heard a voice telling her to come outside. Being a sensible woman, she remained where she was, peering out the window at nothing in the darkness. The next night, the voice came to her again, this time making it clear that she was to build a church. For days following she worried over the means with which she was to accomplish this feat, until it came to her through the words of a Sunday sermon she attended: "God will provide." On the way home, she passed a barn that had blown down from the storm of the night before. Rallying her family, friends, and neighbors, they gathered wood and nails from the fallen structure and, from these, built a church—a small, white church on a neatly landscaped lot. And as we stood in front of it talking, no car passed on the highway without a wave of acknowledgment.[32]

These are the kinds of women that made good midwives: they had magical qualities, and the community knew it. They were called upon for other healing remedies as well; for the midwife was their doctor. "My mother was a granny woman for about all of th' community. They come after her 'cause she was their doctor. People'd come after her, and she'd just always go. They just depended on her same as th' doctor."[33]

No matter how the state regarded the midwife, she commanded her own community's highest respect. "Folks had a lot of confidence in them."[34] She was the local wise woman who presided over the important occasion of birth. She was divinely called (in most cases) and the bearer of a family legacy. She was a trusted leader of her community.

> Yeah, she [her mother] was there that night when mine was born, and then I was there when hers was born. Aunt Martie Harrison delivered her baby. She was a blind woman. Yeah, she delivered my second 'un. With mine she's just as good, though. Sometimes the doctor would get tangled up, you know, get up against somethin' in deliverin' babies that way; and they'd always send for Mis' Harrison. She'd go do the work. Everybody thought more of her than they did the doctor about deliverin' babies. [Laughter.][35]

Not everyone thought so highly of the midwife. The state's health experts would view her leadership as a problem to be circumvented, and her craft as a menace to the public health.

Chapter Two

Public Health Menace

The State's View of the Midwife

Midwives and the State of Florida

Time was in Florida (1927) when, should you *wish* to be registered as a midwife, you simply went down to the office of the circuit court and entered your name and address under the section entitled "Physicians, Midwives, Sextons, Retail Casket Dealers, and Undertakers." But in 1931, with the passage of Florida's first midwifery law, that was all going to change. Now one would need to be licensed in order to practice, and to be licensed, one needed to meet a few conditions: specifically, to be able to read the manual for midwives and to fill out a birth certificate—i.e., to be literate—and to attend fifteen births under the supervision of a licensed, registered physician.

The state had been involved with the midwives long before the passage of the law. In 1915, the Florida State Board of Health experimented with the supervision of midwives by employing four traveling general health nurses, each covering a region of the state. And in 1918, Dr. Grace Whitford established the Bureau of Education and Child Welfare, from which she conducted the first midwifery classes held in the state. In the early 1920s, after receiving Sheppard-Towner[1] funds, the traveling nurses began distributing silver nitrate drops for the prevention of blindness in newborns and doing "investigations" of the midwives' homes. These inspections of home and method were said to have caused five hundred midwives to quit their trade in 1924. By 1926, 3,018 classes were held around the state with 9,966 midwives reported in attendance.[2]

With passage of the new law, efforts toward the regulation of the midwife were intensified. And the first step in controlling the midwives was to find them. It was estimated in 1933 that at least one-third of the births in Florida were midwife attended and that the number of midwives practicing approached four thousand.[3] To build a comprehensive list of potential licensing candidates, the board of health sent a letter to women who were known to be practicing, requesting that they register with their respective county health departments. The midwives' response was immediate and overwhelming. In good faith and from an earnest desire to have their work legally recognized, 630 midwives, out of the 1,400 contacted, voluntarily and without further provocation turned in their names for regulation by the state. A state health official commented, "We were all amazed at the results of this campaign." Not knowing if the remaining eight hundred were offending the law on purpose or through ignorance, the official concluded, "I do believe that in the course of time we will be able to eliminate them."[4]

While many physicians, on record, reflected racist attitudes in the extreme, there were some state bureaucrats who exhibited a milder form of racism in their patronizing attitude. David K. Fulton's report on Florida's "midwife problem," entitled "A Long Dark Night," is typical (see appendix). Coupling a short-story format with factual reporting, Fulton focuses his report around Mattie, a "typical," but fictional, Florida midwife in the year 1910. The overriding tone of the piece is dreary, featuring all of midwifery's darkest sides and little else. In contradiction to the midwife's superior statistics, Mattie, in just sixteen pages of narrative, loses two mothers and their babies, while success-fully delivering but one—the one delivery about which we receive no details. Contemplating the day's calamities, Mattie thinks, "Well, three alive in a row, that was pretty good." Fulton goes on to say, "Mattie wanted to catch them all alive and healthy, but she never got past six or seven, and then would come a bad day, and her heart would be heavy." Unfortunately, the only person in the story *not* based on fact is the main character herself, Mattie—a disturbing factor, considering the report's accountability in determining the future livelihood of real-life midwives. All others, "identified as workers for the public health agen-cies, are true characters, and their words and actions are paraphrased only because no 'sound on film' camera was on the scene." The testi-mony of public health workers—people like David Fulton—weighs heavier than the testimony of the midwives themselves. While apolo-getic, even regretful, for having to paraphrase the words of bureau-crats, he deems unimportant the actual opinions and experiences of the midwives, about whom policies are being made.

Like many of his colleagues, Fulton ascribes to his "fictional mid-wife" the well-worn attributes of uncleanliness, superstition, and ig-norance.

> The last few foraging roaches scurried for the darkness as Mattie pulled a greasy brown dress over her head. Her morning toilet thus completed, she shuffled to the stove. . . . There was a barbeque tonight, and the white ladies had told Mattie that she must wear a clean white dress, and shoes, and a cap. Mattie knew what clean meant, and knew that it meant she would have to wash today.

After painting shadows across Mattie's personal hygiene, Fulton ap-plies his dismal brush to her personal character as well.

> Mattie had come home late one night and found a man waiting for her in her house. The two had been known to be casual friends, and Mattie was said by some to have acted as though she were willing for the relationship

to progress. No one knew the details, but the man was found the next day where he had crawled some distance from Mattie's house, so battered that it appeared he might not make it. He did, but from then on no man, and very few women, bothered to ask Mattie why she remained unmarried.

Fulton does not appear to base his character on direct personal experience with any one midwife but calls his creation a composite—one, no doubt, of his worst nightmares. His biases are confirmed in the character of Dr. Scott, the story's representative physician, who shines like a saint next to poor ol' ignorant Mattie. Dr. Scott expresses a mild, righteous frustration at the conditions of Mattie's practice but generously does not blame *her* for it. In parting, the charitable fellow makes this offer: "Mattie, if you've got one coming along and you think she's going to have trouble, get her into town somehow and let me see her. I won't charge if she hasn't any money." After reading this, one begins to doubt whether Fulton had had any direct experience with doctors, as well. In the style of the true professional elitist, Fulton guffaws at the midwife's apprenticeship training, comparing it to learning how to swim "after a fashion by thrashing about to keep from drowning." With a total disregard for factual information and a slant that betrays an indifference to the real-life women he has just slandered, Fulton concludes his report with this:

> Our history, that portion of our work which constitutes the final section of each chapter, will be that of the midwife control and education program of the Florida State Board of Health, not the history of the midwives themselves. The latter, though more exotic than statistical tables, exists only in remembered anecdote, and hardly lends itself to serious compilation for any worthy purpose.

Fulton's indifference to facts and his penchant for assumption spills over into other similar reports of that period, as in the preface of "Midwifery in Florida."[5] No factual data supports that document's statement that midwives were the prime reason for Florida's one-in-ten infant death rate. "The dirt, ignorance and superstition of early midwifery will not be belabored in this work," because it is already assumed in the minds of both the writer and his audience. And a Pennsylvania doctor's description of Florida as "a capital setting for Dante's Inferno" does not warrant equating midwifery with other "environmental vexations" like hog cholera, yellow fever, and malaria. It is faulty logic to infer that because there was a midwifery program, there must have existed a "serious problem" *with the midwives.*

Studies showed that physicians were in no better position than immigrant midwives when it came to introducing infection at childbirth.[6] In fact, midwives were less likely to encounter childbed fever because of their noninterventive approach in labor and the homogeneous bacterial environment of home delivery. The hospital, as a harbor for the sick, exposed mother and child to a cross section of foreign bacteria, placing them at greater risk for puerperal fever. The application of asepsis, in childbirth as well as in other forms of health care, was a relatively recent development in American history.[7] Only since 1885 has antisepsis been hospital policy, and even up to the 1930s and 1940s puerperal fever was still a danger due to carelessness in hospital antiseptic routine, for example, sterilizing a needle by running it through a bar of soap. Asepsis came to the outreaches of Florida only a short time later, and certainly there were extreme cases of poor conditions, but the middle-class white professional's correlation of filth with poverty is not always and everywhere the case. In other words, it is possible to use old newspapers to patch the holes in one's wall to make do and still maintain a neat and clean home; a well-meaning health official, however, might not find it so when comparing it to his own more comfortable environs.

Another factor to consider is the comparative quality of obstetrical education during this period. J. Whitridge Williams conducted a survey in 1911 of American obstetrical schools in which he discovered more than one-third of the professors to be general practitioners. Thirteen of the professors had seen less than five hundred cases of labor; five, less than one hundred; and one had never witnessed a birth before becoming a professor. Eleven of the professors did not think their graduates were "competent to practice obstetrics."[8] Williams, winner of his alma mater's obstetric prize, had himself only *observed* two deliveries before graduating in 1888.[9] By comparison, 40 percent of New York City's midwives possessed European diplomas, which generally required more extensive training (Swedish and Italian midwives attended one hundred supervised deliveries before certification).[10] And black midwives in the South had shown themselves eager for advanced training when courses were offered (some walked eight to ten miles just to get to class). Still, physicians coupled concentration on improvements in medical education with the elimination of the midwives, whom they denounced as impossible to reeducate. And when faced with the facts of surveys like Williams's they responded, "*A priori* the replies seem to indicate that women in labor are as safe in the hands of admittedly ignorant midwives as in those of poorly educated medical men. Such a conclusion, however, is contrary to reason." While rational *reasons* were seldom advanced in developing a plan to erase the midwife's occupation, a rational *method* was applied with results devastating to the midwife.

There did exist public health workers who earnestly sought to better the midwife without an eye toward her elimination. But overall, the most a midwife could hope to evoke in the average official was a wary condescension and never the full respect she received from her community. Perhaps the health officials just proffered their own brand of respect; one surgeon suggested having "respect for the 'Grannys' but caution not to be contaminated by them."[11] Some had a time mustering up even that much: "They [the midwives] are too dumb, I can't waste my time on them," complained a Florida county public health nurse. To which Nurse Ely replied, "It does take patience to accomplish things with midwives. . . . The midwives are teachable even though they are illiterate and do many things we wish they wouldn't. Still you can get a certain amount of results from them."[12] Even a midwife proponent, New York physician T. J. Hill, envisioned the midwife to "sit at the feet of her Gamaliel [the physician] and hearken to his admonitions on things pertaining to the art of obstetrics."[13]

The midwife had a definite image problem. Dr. O. R. Thompson of Macon, Georgia, declared Southern midwives more difficult to train than Northern because the former were primarily "ignorant" and "superstitious" blacks.[14] At a 1982 legislative hearing on Florida's current midwifery statute, the obstetricians' representative made a loose comparison between legislating midwife-attended home births and regulating the voodoo practice of sacrificing chickens.[15] The midwife was reduced to "an amply proportioned Aunt Jemima, quick of mind, jovial of mood, and of great stature in the community."[16] And as Fulton accurately reflected, "those who carry on her work today look back with scornful eye upon the tribal rites she commemorated in her practice."

One state supervisory nurse complained of the public's ignorance of "the problem" and the lack of cooperation from local municipal governments to enforce the law. She admitted that the law alone would not bring control into effect. Only public opinion would do it, and those interested would have to work to "create an opinion."[17] Nurse Ely told of her efforts to enlighten an enquiring Tampa policeman who saw a large group of midwives assembled for one of the midwife institutes. She showed him a picture of a blind girl who didn't get her silver nitrate drops at birth; of a man who delivered two hundred babies over thirty-five years, having learned how by delivering sows; and she told him of a *black* man who had delivered a *white* woman—both mother and baby died of tetanus. Although there were only seven known male midwives in the state of Florida, it is interesting that she chooses to "create an opinion" about an estimated fifteen hundred women from this isolated group. After relating this "shocking" public ignorance, she pontificated further:

That is just a few of the things that are happening in the state in regard to midwives that many people are not aware of and they think that this condition does not exist. They say that it doesn't exist. One person who seemed interested in the nurses' work I started to tell about the midwife work. She said, "I don't want to see pictures like that—those things are for doctors and nurses." I believe that is too much the attitude of the public in general. They don't want to do anything about it. But the midwife problem is with us today and looms quite large.[18]

Couched in the offended sensibilities of the middle class, the isolated and extreme cases, like the ones cited above, were overzealously used as "reason enough" to make every birth conform to a more professional and calculated standard. This was seen as the *only* remedy. At a 1933 meeting of Florida health officials, Dr. Henry Hanson, the state's public health officer, commented on the lower mortality rates achieved by Florida midwives compared to the higher rates with doctors. And yet he still emphasized lowering the state's high mortality rates by working with the *midwives*. Of course, the physicians did not come under his jurisdiction, but even after training programs in Florida had been established and proven successful, health officials still spoke of the lay midwife's demise as the *ultimate* sign of success.

The hope of the future was the nurse-midwife, as Ethel Kirkland, a Florida public health nursing consultant, suggested in 1973: "When the Certified Nurse-Midwife is fully accepted and her service utilized fully, perhaps there will not be a need to continue to license the lay midwife."[19] The nurse-midwife, an institutionally trained midwife who would work within the hospital structure, was thought to be the compromise. For the traditional midwives, however, it was no compromise; they would lose their right to practice their trade. With no Florida statistics linking high mortality to midwifery and with national statistics placing her above all other attendants in low mortality, still the trend continued: the solution always came around to eliminating the midwife.

Florida's Educational Programs for Midwives

While the black-rich voices of the midwife choir intoned a hymn, the medical director of the Florida Agricultural and Mechanical College (FAMC) gave his notes another once-over. His speech topic: "Why Midwives Should Have Annual Physical Exams"; the choir's selection: "Let Your Will Be Done." It was a prophetic juxtaposition, a caricature of the sometimes uneasy convergence of midwives and state health officials. State and tradition made their first formal introductions at the 1933 West Florida Midwife Institute on the campus of Florida Agricultural and Mechanical College (now FAMU) in Tallahassee.[20] The midwife institute was a state invention to bring midwives from the surrounding regions together for a week of classes on aseptic childbirth attendance. Many came by bus, breaking with their home routines to spend a week in "the city," sharing room, board, and instruction with other midwives like themselves. Although the Tampa area had a large number of white midwives, most photographic records show the majority of institute participants to be older black women. The course offerings ranged from inspections of the midwives' bags[21] to delivery demonstrations on "Miss Chase," the life-size birthing mannequin designed by Jule Graves, the state supervisory nurse overseeing midwives. Except for her trapdoor abdomen, Miss Chase (who came in both black- and whiteface) gave well-simulated births, complete with baby, umbilical cord, and placenta.[22] Still, what the midwives learned from each other during late-night talks *after* class must have rivaled what they learned *in* class. Imagine their excitement in seeing gathered all in one place such a large group of women who, like themselves, had answered the calling of midwifery. Posing for the photographer as solemnly as any graduating class, the midwives were numerous and dignified. And at the week's end, they each carried home a "certificate of fitness," a kind of diploma with no legal significance, which indicated that they had attended classes, had displayed a clean midwife's bag, and "could answer fairly well the questions asked by the nurse."[23] A midwife would usually pin this certificate to her manual, which she carried in her bag when she went on deliveries.[24] There was no legal obligation for midwives to attend the institutes. A woman choosing to forgo them could practice unhampered, but many midwives were glad for the opportunity.

The midwife institutes were periodically organized around the state for thirteen years. Among archive records, a copy of a 23 May 1946 letter announces the permanent discontinuance of the midwife institutes. There began a shift of concentration from state to local supervision; Nurse Kirkland, a state midwife consultant, would be making her rounds across the state, accompanied by a comprehensive slide show.[25] Both midwives and state officials seemed to agree on the institutes' success, but there was concern on the part of the latter over what permanent impression they made without local follow-up. Considering the state's long-term goal of eliminating lay midwifery, it is possible that the midwife institutes were *too* successful. Bringing midwives together from a large area must have produced a sense of strength and solidarity from which they had previously been isolated in their individual communities. Though they came to be instructed in the way the *state* preferred them to attend childbirths, it would have been hard to measure what percentage of knowledge they took from the classes and what percentage was reinforced by fellow classmates. The midwife was freer to pick and choose which policies she would incorporate once she returned home where there was no one looking over her shoulder. Also, the unity and pride the midwives gleaned from the weeklong institutes were counterproductive to persuading them to later forsake their vocations altogether. In short, the midwife institutes provided strength without control. Moving supervisory power to the local level in conjunction with the titular reinforcement of the state more effectively controlled the midwives and proved more compatible with the state's program of elimination. The midwives' awareness of their strength in numbers and vocational integrity was correspondingly diminished.

Even with the passage of the 1931 midwife law, there still existed no provisions for enforcement, causing critics to complain of a statute with "no teeth." State officials were unsuccessful in trying to persuade local authorities to apply the law in respect to certain midwives from local influential families. There was also concern as to how the new law could be implemented in light of the inferior educational opportunities for blacks in Florida. A midwife improvement plan, to be funded by the U.S. Children's Bureau based in Atlanta, was developed to answer this need. Improvement was not directed to the older existing midwives but to younger women just coming up, who were "to serve areas where medical service cannot be secured for Negro women during labor and delivery and [is] now given by 'granny midwives.' "[26] A select number of women from around the state would be housed and instructed at FAMC in Tallahassee for a period of three months. Aside from transportation costs, the state would pick up the bill. During their stay, the midwives were expected to observe five deliveries at the adjoining clinic and attend twenty births. Successful candidates would be sent to organized health departments around the state upon completion of their course of study. After a six-month supervised probationary period in their respective counties each candidate was issued her license if the "health department feels that the trainee should be licensed."[27] This program was open only to black women between the ages of twenty-five and forty-five. Completion of an eighth-grade or equivalent education was required, as well as a physical exam and a letter from the woman's minister vouching for her moral character. A 9 June 1945 letter announced the plan's approval by the Children's Bureau and the promise of funds, but by 23 May 1946 another letter informed an interested party of the plan's discontinuance. Reportedly, the plan could not enlist enough participants to warrant its existence. Few women could afford the cost of transportation from the length of the state, and those who could were unable to leave home, family, and work for such an extended period of time. The age limit, transportation costs, and the unrealistic requirement of the midwife to defer home responsibilities virtually disqualified most if not all of the traditional granny midwives from the program.

Finally, after experimenting with the installment of four or five traveling supervisory nurses over delineated districts, the placement of permanent state representatives in each county became the preferred plan. This was accomplished within each county's existing bureaucratic framework and in the person of the county public health nurse. The nurses were approached individually by state officials, requesting that they incorporate the supervision of midwives into their already existing duties. All but two accepted these added responsibilities and worked with the state supervisory nurse to locally enforce the state's plan. Later, as the county position over the midwives became more institutionalized, the nurses who were sought to fill these posts were "young colored nurse[s] of pleasing personality." These women were usually brought down from the North and were trained by the state nurse to supervise, hold classes, and inspect the midwives' bags. They administered state policies at the local level, and it was thought that their color and youth would be more persuasive to the most resistant of the old midwives. Persuasion was always an important part of the midwife plan. Forcing compliance to the new law on the old midwives was sometimes difficult because of the midwife's entrenched status within her own community. Less than honest means were often employed in this persuasion. Dr. Paul Coughlin's attitude is a case in point: "We will have to talk to the old 'grannies' and coax them into thinking that they are helping to train the new ones. The old midwives will still retain their cases and receive their fees, but the students will do a considerable portion of the work."[28]

One of the county nurse's responsibilities was to preside over monthly midwife club meetings. The meetings' ostensible function was instruction; the county nurse would advise the midwives of new rules, show displays, do bag inspections, and discuss the high risks of attending mothers with high blood pressure, syphilis, gonnorhea, or herpes, as well as instruct them in anatomy and delivery with an emphasis on noninterference. One midwife said they seldom learned anything new at these meetings, "just how to make beds and shave 'em [the mothers])," but all the same, "us loves our meetings!" Many midwives spoke of their fondness for these gatherings as much for their social and supportive qualities as anything else. For the state, they were a monitoring device through which the county nurse could closely supervise the midwives, ensuring their observance of state policy. Meanwhile, the state supervisory nurse traveled the state, consulting with the county nurses and holding one-day classes for the licensed midwives—the format of the new institute. These coincided with the regular monthly midwife meetings. The state nurse appeared *with* the county nurse to ensure "uniformity" of state and county policy. And it was at these meetings that the conflict between the state's requirements and the midwife's calling was most acute. The midwives were leaders in their communities and not prone to take things lying down, and when the edicts of the state were in disaccord with the tenets of their calling, compliance to "the rules" could be trying. A major area of contention was the health departments' efforts to circumscribe the midwife's clientele. Public health personnel advised her to refuse service to a woman who did not have the doctor's permit, which certified a woman for a midwife-attended birth. The midwife was encouraged to adopt a plan of payment for her services that required the client to make advance monthly installments during pregnancy. This posed a moral dilemma for the midwife, who felt herself called by God to share her gift regardless of the circumstances.

> Mrs. White recommends that they obtain payment in advance, taking the stance that the basis of a midwife-client relationship is structured, formal, and businesslike, likening it to the doctor-patient relationship. Speaking to

a midwife, but not directly to the nurse, one midwife states that they are all "Christian women," obligated to serve women in need. It is God's will that they serve, whether women intend to pay them or not, pointing out the essential element of selfless service in traditional midwifery. Midwives are *bound* to serve and have status related to supernatural sanctions.[29]

Licensure of Midwives

Licensing was a bureaucratic device for control. It determined the standards by which women could practice midwifery, who would be allowed to practice, and who would be barred. Florida's 1931 statute delegated licensing power to the Florida State Board of Health. At first the object was to enroll as many midwives as possible into the program, or in the process to at least identify who was practicing. The names of the first midwife registrants were gathered from local registrars in 1930 and were used to promote the enactment of Florida's midwifery law. Out of 107 white and 840 "colored" registrants, 102 white and 714 black women were licensed.[30] Licenses were not granted to some for reasons of old age, minimal practice, syphilis, and/or failure to enlist the recommendations of two doctors. Midwives were allowed to continue only in areas where they did not compete with existing medical facilities. These areas were limited to predominantly black populations, and further narrowed to rural blacks. It was never the state's objective to enhance the midwife profession. Midwives would be tolerated where the poor needed care, but only until that situation could be corrected. In the meantime, the number of licensed midwives steadily diminished from year to year, until the board of health's 1963 annual report boasted twelve counties without midwives. By 1942, with the admission of three young black nurses into a six-month midwifery course, an emphasis was put on the retirement of old midwives. And these were to be replaced "with nurse-midwives who can more intelligently carry on this phase of the work."[31] That year's state midwife consultant reported her success in urging fifteen granny midwives to end their practices. In 1968 the public health nurse could report with even greater pride that not one new applicant applied for a midwife's license. This "accomplishment" was, no doubt, a direct result of a 1965 provision that required applicants to first establish need before being accepted as trainees. Recommendations from a local private physician and the public health officer provided this proof of need. With the expansion of modern medical facilities and with the number of physicians increasing, it was most difficult to get such recommendations, especially when the midwife was considered a primitive form to be eradicated.

In the end, the midwife program's greatest feat was working itself out of a job. The state had finally met its objective when there were no longer midwives to license. This came about in as many ways as there were counties. Though the criteria for licensure were a matter of state statute, the unwritten and eventual goal was to phase out lay midwifery altogether. And each county nurse, within the law's parameters, was given wide range in the accomplishment of this end while carrying out her ostensible duties of training and supervision. This local authority was especially enhanced when Works Progress Administration funds were halted, forcing the state board of health to reorganize and allot more power to each community. After more counties established individual health units, decentralization was emphasized in 1947 with responsibility shifted to county health units. The varying speed with which each county accomplished the phaseout of the traditional midwife depended on indigenous factors, not the least of which was the extent of hospital facilities and the number of practicing physicians in place. It also depended on the personal attitudes of the county nurse toward the midwife and, when these were unfavorable, the ferocity with which she exercised her office. In neighboring counties, a midwife's loss of an infant during birth might have two different consequences, depending on the county nurse's handling of the situation. One county nurse was notorious for her unyielding position on midwives, recommending to state officials—without a hearing or regard for the midwife's practice record—license revocation of a midwife who had delivered over five hundred babies.[32] Since there were no uniform standards for age or disciplinary measures for mishandled cases, retirement and revocation were matters determined somewhat arbitrarily by each county nurse, though procedures went through the state office.

A conflict in values was at the base of the relationship between the midwives and the health department. Though many of the midwives' skills may have been improved by the institutes and educational programs, the antagonism residing in the state's true regard and intention for the midwife could not help but surface. In the beginning of the midwife improvement program, the state health nurse's annual reports showed pleasure in the growing numbers of midwives attending the institutes and coming forward to be licensed. In the later years, there was just as much excitement for their decline. "Efforts to improve and extend medical services to all maternity patients have been rewarded as evidenced by the fact that licensed midwives are not practicing in eighteen counties."[33] The measure of the program's success was not in the refinement of the midwife's skills but in her decreasing numbers. Health officials worked hard to better the midwife and to provide her with educational opportunities, but it was for the purpose of control aimed toward elimination. Her personal dignity and respect for her occupation were secondary concerns, when they were considered at all.

Chapter Three

The Uneasy Meeting of Tradition and State

Phaseout of the Midwives

They didn't have t'have a license when they first began, as far back as I can remember. I didn't know of 'em havin' t'have 'em until up later years. Then they got t'where if they delivered babies, they had t'have a license. And then they were finally just completely cut out of th' job at all. Weren't allowed to'do th' job at all.[1]

When the first midwives voluntarily registered their names with the state of Florida, they unknowingly began a chain of events that would lead to the demise of their trade. They bequeathed to their daughters and granddaughters not only their calling but a struggle for the right to practice it. They believed that the state was taking a positive interest in their contributions by providing them, for the first time, with legal recognition and training for the refinement of their craft. Certainly they did not know of physicians like J. Clifton Edgar of New York, who regarded them as an "evil" to be "eradicated" and who promoted licensing and training as a temporary measure to minimize the midwife's threat to the public.[2] Nor would they have guessed the real reason behind such liberal licensing standards, according to which people like Dr. S. W. Newmayer were advising officials to grant as many licenses as possible as a means of monitoring the midwives with an eye toward their eventual elimination.[3] This was preferable to allowing them to go undetected and unsupervised.

Two state programs were consistent with and instrumental in accelerating the phaseout process. In the earlier years of midwife improvement, when midwives were still a Southern necessity, the long-term goal was to replace the granny midwife with the nurse-midwife. The latter would service the same clientele as the granny but with a formal education that provided her with an orientation more compatible with the existing medical structures. The "voluntary" honorable discharge was an apparatus through which this transition was made. It accomplished an unpleasant task in the most benign style thought possible by "retiring" the aging midwife with a banquet and ceremony in her honor. Prior to this occasion, she would be enlisted in helping the county nurse to select her replacement, who would "follow in her footsteps" (that is, when she was not in class).

> The State Board of Health advocates that the retiring midwife sell her equipment to her young protégé—thereby removing the temptation to take an occasional case. When arrangements have been completed and the young midwife is ready, a ceremony is conducted at the monthly midwife meeting. At this meeting the retiring midwife asks for an "honorable discharge" from her county midwife club, and signs a card promising not to accept any more cases. She then becomes an *ex officio* member of the local midwife club. This procedure removes the possibility of needlessly hurting her feelings, as she feels that she is not simply discarded. The other midwives know that she has voluntarily resigned.[4]

That was the state's view of it. To Mary Beth Chambers, recipient of a certificate of honorable discharge, there was nothing voluntary about her resignation. Neither were there any fools among her midwife colleagues who thought otherwise.

I ain't told 'em, no; I wasn't the one told 'em I was gonna retire. They just called it retirement, 'cause I don't know nothin' *'bout* no retirement. I thought as far as retirement is concerned, it'd be you know it when you get in it, don't ya? A certain age you retire? A certain time? That was never mentioned, nothin' like that. But, as I told you, she just tol' me. One day I went in there, I had somethin' or other before them, she said, "You about ready to retire?" I said, "Well, if I have to, I will. I just [left it kinda light]. . . . And so many places they was cuttin' out the midwives anyhow. So I thought they wanted 'em out of G—— County, too.

Mrs. Chambers's description of her "retirement" ceremony also makes it clear that the state's duplicity, even disguised in a benign farewell ceremony, was still quite evident to midwives displaced from their lifelong profession.

Well, Miss M—— [county health nurse] was the one, and the doctor—I can't think of his name—he was there. They had all of the midwives in there, and they just had a talk and dinner, and then they asked me to say whatever I desired to say—a word or two. . . . Well, I thanked 'em for appreciating me enough to have the luncheon *with* me, and I let 'em know that I enjoyed workin' with them, and if it was the rule for me to retire at this time, well, I would accept it. But I let 'em know *definitely* that I didn't know any too much about it, and they never just said directly. 'Cause she the one that asked me; said she couldn't sign another license. Wouldn't be capable for her to sign another license. I had delivered [only] about three or four babies [that year]. And so I put it to that, and then I heard after then, it was that and the age. But *she* didn't tell me.[5]

Meeting Mrs. Chambers three years later, when she was seventy-seven, I found her to be alert of mind and movement and younger in appearance than her age revealed. But older midwives, however young in mind and spirit, could not have their licenses renewed if no births were attended over a two-year period. Some midwives complained of not knowing this stipulation until it was too late, and others, like Mrs. Chambers, reported having attended two or three babies within the year they were retired. This policy was a Department of Health and Rehabilitative Services (HRS) invention and not a clause in the Florida statute; it provided an excuse for expediting the phaseout ahead of schedule. County health policies abetted the reduction of the midwife's practice and then penalized her for a diminished clientele. No similar age restrictions or minimum quotas were applied to physicians, who could practice as long as *they* deemed fit. Age limitations for midwives were determined arbitrarily by health officials whose rationales had as much to do with the phaseout plan's progress as with the public's well-being. "We do have a district for Mary Etta Shelby. Janie Jones, who is our most prominent midwife here in Pensacola, has been recommended for retirement by Dr. Marsh, due to her age ⟨70 years of age)."[6]

Another device that facilitated the phaseout of the midwives was the doctor's permit, described by a Miami doctor as a "distinct advance" in the control of the midwife. This was a pledge card, requiring a physician's signature, that certified low-risk mothers for midwife-attended births while serving as a sort of contract between the midwife and her client. The client agreed to obey the midwife, and the midwife promised to see that her client got prenatal care from a doctor or the county clinic. It was an effective method for enlisting compliance with the law from the public as well as from the midwife and, as it turned out, served to proselytize clients for the hospital.[7] After making their prenatal visits at a county clinic or hospital, some women, when it was financially feasible, chose to forgo their midwives and have their deliveries there as well. And in the 1960s, with the availability of federal health care funds to the poor coupled with desegregation legislation, this trend became more pronounced. As hospital facilities became more accessible, the permits were granted less frequently by physicians who were unwilling to recommend mothers for home births. More than ever, the hospital was viewed as the only sensible place to have a baby. The definition of high-risk was broadened, and everything from high blood pressure to youthful pregnancies was now deemed unfit for home birth. Evelyn Reynolds described this situation as it developed with her mother, Georgia Reynolds:

> She began to sense that something was going on. At first, she thought it was a good thing that she could go up to the clinic and meet her mothers up there. And a lot of times, she . . . would go and pick up four and five women who didn't have transportation, carry them to meet the maternity clinic, and help them to weigh them, working *with* the staff. This is the type of thing that she *thought* was a betterment for all concerned. But as it worked out, she found out a lot of her clients—clients she had delivered four and five babies for—were beginning to tell her, "Well, Mis' Reynolds, Mis' A—— is telling me I need to go to the hospital." And Mother says, "Well, let me get on the phone and talk with her and see if there's any complications setting in. Because if there were, well, it was okay. If they feel like they found somethin' wrong with your blood or something wrong with your urinary system or something, then you *need* to go." But there wouldn't be anything wrong with them. She would actually check it out. And what happened, they would attend this clinic, and eventually, after attending so many times—I think they went like once a month or once every two weeks—they would give them a card stating that they were alright for midwifery delivery and more or less okay from the clinic. And all of a sudden Mama wasn't getting cards. . . . No one is giving you any feedback as to *why* it's happening, but you see it happening. It got to the place that Mother's ward was just catching dust, and I seen the time the calendar was just lined *up* with babies being born. She had two delivery rooms, as I said, and those delivery rooms were hot; she kept them busy from one to the other having a baby. . . . She just got to the place where she just sat there and she looked at her equipment—no deliveries, no one coming. And she got, well, I would say, at first, she got a little angry about it. This type of thing, someone killing your career, is just like killing some member of the family that's real close. At first, she began to wonder. You ask yourself questions: "Well, what have *I* done wrong?" You look back, and you say, "I've delivered maybe thirty or forty babies on the average of a month for years. And I've only lost one mother, and that mother was lost

in a hospital with the doctor attending." And you haven't had that many stillbirths, and you begin to wonder, "Well, what in the world am I doing wrong? . . ." No one is giving any answers on it. So you just pretty soon feel whipped. . . . She just kept sittin' there lookin' at her equipment collect dust, and she'd go by and make the beds up, just hopin' things would get better. And they didn't ever get any better.[8]

As late as the 1980s there still remained, usually in the rural areas, midwives who survived these programs with a small clientele. To close in on the midwife's practice even further, attention was turned once again to the midwife's clients. Rigid boundary lines, irrespective of county jurisdictions, were drawn up, disallowing the midwife to cross over into communities she may have once served. In Gadsden, the northern Florida county that boasts the most traditional midwives still practicing, a midwife could serve both Jackson and Liberty counties but not adjoining Leon County. The reason given for the hands-off policy in Leon was that "follow-up is a problem." Since the Gadsden County midwives were allowed to cross not only these county lines but the state line of Georgia, it would seem unlikely that follow-up was the reason. Until 1979, Leon County sustained one hospital obstetric unit, which engendered not a small amount of controversy over what some called its monopolistic tendencies.[9] In recent years, several young women in Tallahassee had sought to have their home births *legally* with a *licensed* midwife. Gadsden County was the home of the nearest licensed lay midwife, but she was not allowed to make the thirty-minute drive into Leon County to make a delivery. The young mothers, however, were allowed to cross into Gadsden provided they fulfilled two criteria: they had to take all their prenatal examinations at the Gadsden County Health Department, and they would be required to present a doctor's permit recommending them as low-risk mothers. While the first stipulation was bothersome, the second was virtually impossible. Fearing revocation of hospital privileges and malpractice insurance, few, if any, doctors would sign such a card.[10] This served as an effective obstruction to the union of the rural granny midwife with the middle-class mother of the home-birth movement—a meeting that would have opened up a whole new pool of clients for the midwife's sagging career.

Midwives found that allowing state control of their practices entitled related agencies to become involved as well. Some of these were consciously and quite legally used to pressure midwives into quitting. The use of county code-enforcement agencies was especially effective in urban black areas where buildings were run down or substandard. And some urban midwives, in order to manage numerous cases more conveniently, ran maternity homes in these areas. The homes were set up for food and laundry service and thus were also subject to municipal sanitation codes. Inspections of the maternity homes, in some cases, were used as tools of harassment. Periodic visits from various agencies (e.g., fire safety, building code) proved effective means in closing down the homes. This was the case of one Florida midwife (also a licensed practical nurse) who, having suffered the same woes the doctor's permit had brought to Mrs. Reynolds, had still managed to keep her maternity home open.[11] Code-enforcement officers began their inspections, forcing the home to close until violations were corrected. Once reopened, another inspection took place, new violations were cited, and so it went. The midwife's clients could no longer depend on the home and naturally diminished in number to the point where it was no longer feasible to stay open.

County building codes were also used against Mrs. Stephenson's efforts to attend women in her rural home, a sensible solution for an older midwife who no longer relished the extensive travel required in her younger days. Mrs. Stephenson built an addition to her home that was to serve as a birthing room. After the building was completed, the county nurse advised her not to use the room until the county's building code requirement of an extra bathroom was met. The midwife was not financially able to tackle another expenditure so soon and was forced to be content with fewer clients.

Yet another government agency to contribute to the midwife's demise was the federal welfare system. Low-cost hospital plans for the poor were first mentioned in the 1957 annual report of the Florida State Board of Health. These were provided through municipal and private agencies and enabled the low-income patient to be delivered at the hospital. Some offered a prepayment plan that allowed the patient to pay her hospital bill in small weekly installments. In later years, what remained of the midwife's clientele were mostly poor women unable to pay for the expensive services of doctor and hospital. The result of these low-cost maternity plans on the midwife's practice was predictable. "Midwives in rural areas are being eliminated where local physicians and hospitals are able to care for indigent prenatals."[12] With the addition of federal subsidies for maternity care to the poor, many of the midwife's clients became aware of welfare benefits that offered to pay all medical costs for those who qualified. Total reimbursement of federal monies would be made to recognized care-givers—the midwife not being one of them. This depleted the midwife's practice mightily and was cited by more than one midwife as a major factor in the final eclipse of midwifery.

> The girls will tell ya, "Miss Rosalind, we don't need you no more. I'm on welfare, and the welfare pay for my baby." See, they won't bill us midwives if us waitin' on one. . . . Only way we get a chance to wait on anyone is just like if a grandmother gonna pay for her daughter if she got pregnant. Now, that's the po' grandmother got to pay, and she haven't been on welfare. But just as quick as that baby born, then she [the mother] go get on welfare. . . . So if I had to just, say, live on what I catch babies, I'd have been dead.[13]

Mrs. Seeley suggested that the inclusion of licensed midwives in these federal provisions might have substantially reduced welfare expenditures since the cost of a midwife's services is less than that of the doctor's. She generously credited this lack of common sense to administrative oversight.[14]

The Midwives' Reactions

Like the midwives who voluntarily registered themselves in the beginning, the latter-day midwives were just as respectful of the law once their licenses were revoked. "I don't deliver no babies. I haven't delivered a baby—that was in '80, and I haven't delivered a baby since, and I will not because I don't have no license."[15] Whether it was from respect, trust, or fear, the midwives showed a desire to work *with* the public health system in providing the best care for all concerned. That their cooperation was not only betrayed but, in fact, enlisted to aid in their own destruction generated feelings of confusion, disappointment, and bitterness. Like Mrs. Reynolds, many midwives looked first to themselves in trying to sort out the reasons for such treatment. They examined their long practices for any flaw that might have offended. The midwives generally held the public health nurses and doctors in high esteem if only because of their superior formal education. "She felt betrayed by the state," explained Mrs. Reynolds's daughter Evelyn. "She knew that the state was behind it. But I think she felt, 'Well, here they are. They've got more education than I have, they have more trainin' than I have, they're sayin' that this is the way it should be done. They're not tellin' me why. This is just it.' "[16]

Though some public health workers, like Jule O. Graves, worked hard to avoid the hurt feelings that were inevitable in the phaseout process, many midwives recalled harsh treatment from nurses and particularly physicians.[17] Mrs. Wilson opened her interview by mentioning the name of a doctor who had told her that he hated the midwives. And every county seemed to have at least one official who viewed it his or her public duty to see to it personally that the midwives be outlawed. Mrs. Jones talked about a doctor who said that there "wadn't no midwives where he come from, and when he leave here, there wadn't gonna be none here." When she boasted to her county nurse of delivering eighteen babies in a month, the nurse replied, "Well, you won't do that again." Mrs. Jones said she didn't know at the time what the nurse meant but remembers that it made her "feel bad."[18] Until the state's objective became clear, the midwives were confused by the health department's ostensible show of support, and all the while it was becoming harder and harder to practice in spite of them. All the midwives were aware of the doctors' exorbitant fees and expressed amazement at what they charged for "just normal baby deliverin'." Some were bitter that some of these same doctors had a hand in limiting the midwife's fee. Three midwives' experiences with public health officials were so bad that they identified my interest in them with yet another state ruse or entrapment, and refused to even consider an interview. One asked, as she walked away, "What do the *midwives* get out of it?"

In the end, midwives generally responded to the phaseout in two ways. Many found that the health department's pressure on them began to outweigh the enjoyment they had once found in their practices. They voluntarily turned in their licenses. Others continued practicing, but with circumspect regard for whatever requests or changes came down from the county or state office. Mrs. Stephenson got wise to the county's use of granny midwives for the training of their own replacements.

> I'll tell you just like I told them: why am I gonna train you, and I'm already knowin' you turnin' me off? I ain't gonna help train you nothin'. That's the way *I* am. They get over there—wanta go out with us on a case. 'Cause I ain't carryin' [them] out with me. They tellin' me they gonna turn us off. And these girls us training are gonna take us place. Let the hospitals train 'em. Let 'em be trained to the hospital.[19]

The midwives were confused as to why their accomplishments and long years of service did not seem to count for much and why, after attending a couple of thousand births, the health department would require them to earn a two-year degree, of which only twenty-two out of sixty-five hours pertained directly to obstetrics. They were hurt that the county health officials, with whom they had worked in such close cooperation and friendship over the years, would betray them. And, offering their own testimonies before legislative hearings on the *new* midwifery law, for a short time they were hopeful that these young, middle-class midwives with their home-birth movement might have just the clout needed to turn things around.

The Co-opting of a Tradition

Just as HRS was closing the final chapter on the phaseout plan in Florida, a fresh wind from the West revived an interest in midwifery within the middle class, beginning a sort of midwifery renaissance. By the 1960s, the corporate model of specialization was the American standard in most areas of public life. Within the medical profession this trend was mirrored in a shift away from the general practice of the family physician toward the more technically oriented specialist. Public health administrators, in turn, adopted this position as their own, making midwife-attended home birth even more unfathomable to modern sensibilities. And with only 123 midwives licensed in 1970, the HRS questioned whether so few midwives merited an entire statewide program replete with paperwork and staff. The obstetrician's hold on childbirth was secure if not rigidified, and the obstetrics wing became a ripe target for women who viewed birth as a natural human process and sought to regain control as a personal right. Midwives were rediscovered as part and parcel of home birth.

Reflective of this rediscovery was a group of "long-haired vegetarians" who moved east from California in 1971 to start a self-sufficient farming community in Summertown, Tennessee, called the Farm. Aside from being the oldest and largest existing commune of its kind in the United States, its real claim to fame was its comprehensive lay midwifery service and neonatal clinic—something that has brought it both national and international prominence. As outlined in Ina May Gaskin's book *Spiritual Midwifery*, the Farm emphasized the emotional and spiritual aspects of childbirth as they occurred in the midwife-attended home setting. A great deal of respect and attention was bestowed on the mother during her pregnancy, and midwife-attended birth was considered a family event and constitutional right.

> We feel that returning the major responsibility for normal childbirth to well-trained midwives rather than have it rest with a predominantly male and profit-oriented medical establishment is a major advance in self-determination for women. The wisdom and compassion a woman can intuitively experience in childbirth can make her a source of healing and understanding for other women.[20]

The Farm midwives' veneration for birth is reflected in their magnanimous offer at the end of *Spiritual Midwifery*. They invite women considering abortion to have their babies at the Farm, where the child would be raised and returned to the mother should she ever want him or her back. This brought a flood of clients from outside the commune who enabled Farm midwives to quickly compile an impressive set of statistics. The area's medical community, unable to ignore the midwives' successful results, provided backup to the clinic and was caught more than once extolling the Farm's midwifery services. Simultaneous with the persuasive book's popularity, and perhaps in part because of it, vital statistics began showing an increase in midwife-attended births as well as births by unnamed attendants. The home-birth movement created a renaissance of midwifery. It was a movement composed largely of the white, youthful middle class, who brought with them the "keys to the board room" that the elderly black women did not have; the education, color, and financial means of their caste made them harder to dismiss by those in power. It looked as though the midwife's luck was about to change.

When young women began applying for the lay midwifery license, the public health officials and local physicians met them head-on with their first impasse: medical backup. Applicants were finding it difficult to secure the required two physicians to sponsor their applications for licensure. And public health officials were also adamant in blocking their progress—some having publicly announced their intentions to never, under any circumstance, license another midwife. Who would have predicted that after years of bureaucratic struggle and planning, a resurgence of interest would occur in, of all places, the scientifically grounded middle class? And things had been going so well; a definition of nurse-midwife was included in 1971 in the rules and regulations for the practice of midwifery, and an enabling act for nurse-midwives was attached to the Nurse Training Act of 1975.[21] And by this time the number of granny midwives practicing in the state was below fifty, while the ranks of the nurse-midwives continued to swell. The long-awaited transition from lay midwives to nurse-midwives was running smoothly, until now. Things were not going as planned.

The new lay midwife applicants answered this opposition with public pressure and court petitions. In 1979 and 1981, in two separate cases, the 1931 law was thrown out as obsolete and thus unconstitutional. One judge cited the law unconstitutional due to vagueness and because delegation of its licensing power by the legislature to HRS violated the state constitution.[22] A Tampa judge also cited it for vagueness, arguing that it did not indicate what kind of conduct was prohibited: "The law requires that a lay midwife be licensed. But it does not define midwife nor does it spell out what actions a midwife performs, leaving those definitions to the Florida Department of Health and Rehabilitative Services."[23] And so it happened that the law, styled to facilitate the occupational phaseout of a portion of the American population, was legally exposed. And until a new law could be drafted, applicants were permitted to write their own lay midwifery licensing examination.

When the 1982 midwifery law was passed at the instigation of the midwife's new middle-class supporters, the apprenticeship model was virtually discarded. In its place were three years of formal training in a course of study that led to eligibility. Also, the applicant was to observe twenty-five births and attend twenty-five more under supervision. By comparison, a nurse-midwife took two years of formal training and came out with a master's degree. The lay midwife, for her trouble, received no degree and no credentials. There was another catch; at that time, no midwifery schools existed in Florida. The midwife lobbyists were not elated with their new law, but in light of the medical community's tough opposition (including that from the nursing association), it was the only compromise they could reach. They were given two years to work out the bugs through an advisory committee composed of one nurse-midwife, one physician (obstetrician or family physician practicing obstetrics), two lay midwives, and a state resident representing the public. At the end of the two-year period, the law would come up for sunset review, at which time it would be evaluated and reconsidered for passage on a more permanent basis. The committee worked intensively to draw up guidelines and to open two midwifery schools in the state during this time.

As for the traditional midwife, she was "grandmothered" into the new law and exempt from qualifying under the new requirements, as were midwives with licenses from other countries with equivalent standards. But that was the last consideration the law's makers afforded her. Some unforeseen consequences of the new law were not as kind to the granny midwife's practice, which existed in a cultural context distinct from the new middle-class midwifery. In the fifty years of licensed midwifery in Florida, an important element in the granny midwife's practice was her close working relationship with the local county health unit. The public health department's involvement with the midwife, though overall suspect, did bring with it some benefits. It provided free instruction to the midwives, rather than requiring them to attend formal nursing schools where they would be trained in hospital settings with textbooks that were formulated, in the main, by physicians. This type of education emphasized the abnormal cases of birth and interventive obstetrics—something the lay midwife's service, by definition, did not include. Rather than learn her trade in the isolated setting of the academy, the granny midwife's training was integrated into the community she served and of which she was a part.

Under the new law, women from two classes and two generations fell under one occupational title. In practice the few younger midwives who were licensed under the old law found the county health department's supervision of them uncomfortable if not openly hostile. The old protocols to which the granny midwife had subscribed were not easily superimposed onto the middle-class midwife or her clientele. The county nurse's routine inspection of the mother a few days after delivery did not meet with much cooperation in middle-class suburbs. Unlike the health department's usual clientele, the patients of the new midwife had their out-of-hospital births for reasons of choice, not finances. The home-birth mother, choosing to birth against the mainstream, espoused an ideology of natural birth as a matter between midwife and family. The county nurse's arrival on this idyllic scene was a shocking intrusion.

The young midwives had experienced harassment from the various county health departments as well as opposition from HRS; therefore, their first goal was to revoke the county health department's supervisory role. Since the young midwives had spearheaded the drive for revised legislation, the advisory committee formulated policy responsive to the needs of these younger women. Now the midwives would report directly to the state HRS office in Tallahassee, and the county nurse was obviated. (An attempt in 1982 to place midwifery under the auspices of the Department of Professional Regulations failed, ostensibly for budgetary reasons.)

The granny midwife was adversely affected in several ways by the elimination of her county liaison. With the removal of the county nurse, the several-page document of the new law and its provisions was sent directly to each midwife. To a few isolated, rural midwives, the law's bureaucratic technical jargon alone was enough to impel them to voluntarily turn in their licenses. The county nurse, who usually translated the state's edicts as they came down, was no longer in place. And without interpretation, the new law appeared to be only a maze of red tape and thus yet another assault on the weary midwife profession. The more determined midwives, however, sought out the county nurse to interpret and demonstrate the new requirements. They learned that the new law brought more freedom to their practices, and yet after years of strict "hands-off" policy, some older midwives found this sudden break with the past confusing. The new midwives had fought for and won the legal use of various instruments in labor and delivery. This was a right denied the granny midwife, who was not even allowed to do internal examinations with her bare hands. Now she was encouraged to use a fetascope, take blood pressure, record Apgar readings,[24] and administer oxygen (something a football coach does routinely). But taking a blood pressure reading, without direction, was an ominous and complex undertaking to some traditional midwives. And others balked at the detailed forms they were now required to fill out for each birth.

The county health department had also served, albeit rarely, as a buffer between the midwife and malpractice suits. Through licensure and close supervision, the midwife's services came under the auspices of the county office. But with the elimination of the county as mediator for the midwife, her practice became more vulnerable to lawsuits should any complications occur with one of her clients. The high costs of malpractice premiums were beyond the means of most rural midwives. Some, fearful of losing all that they had worked for, turned in their licenses. Others, wanting to continue their practices, cautiously put all property in their children's names. Again the law had failed to take the granny midwives into consideration and treated them all as one with the middle-class midwives, who were in a better position to resolve these problems. Losing the shelter of the county health office, the granny midwives were suddenly left to fend for themselves.

> I can't tell you nothin' but just how I started to be a midwife and how I'm *so rarin'* to continue to be a midwife, but we got to go by these laws. And if us got to go by them laws, we *need* a doctor or someone to back us up or be behind us. And if I deliver a baby and the baby is not normal, I suppose to rush and carry it to the health department, then they takes over. But no more. They ain't got no more to do with us. Us on us own. . . . If anything come up, no doctor's gonna help you; they can sue you. I'm on and they're off. [Laughter.] 'Cause my husband gone, and I worked too hard for my home, and I ain't gonna let nobody take it.[25]

Many midwives shared similar feelings about their financial vulnerability. "I'll take a chance if we get over this suing proposition," another midwife said. " 'Cause you don't know never when they get there and you be ruined. And I don't have anything. What I have I need 'cause I'm too old to get anything else. I been years and years gettin' this little house, and I'm gonna keep it."[26]

As had happened so many times before, the needs of the old-style midwife were disregarded in the fluster of compromise that shaped the new law. Under legal pressure from the medical community, the new midwives were anxious to gain a legal status that would end the random harassment. In the face of strong medical opposition, the midwife proponents settled for a statute that all but discarded the apprentice model of lay midwifery for the contemporary model of the institutionally educated nurse-midwife. The lay midwife was to be a professional, receiving her clinical instruction not at the knee of a single preceptor, but in the florescent-lighted classrooms of the academy, which ensured uniform prerequisites under faculty control. Having each midwife apprentice under varying personalities with diverse techniques might have been appropriate for a time when adequate medical facilities were lacking. But that method was too messy and unmanageable for the preferred corporate model of modern health care.

Granted, times had changed, and careers no longer evolved from circumstances, but created them. Still, the granny midwife's career had been a perfect organic model that incorporated each phase of the women's personal and community lives. Few women began their practices before the age of thirty—a time usually taken up with the raising of children. But during this time, they often began a relaxed apprenticeship, assisting a licensed midwife when time permitted. When the children were old enough to fend for themselves, the prospective midwife was ready to formalize her apprenticeship, increasing her time commitments to the work. By this point, she had already observed or assisted fifty to a hundred births. Her preceptor would pass down her practice to her protégé as advancing age tapered her activity. And yet, the old midwife would occasionally be invited to assist the younger midwife on a birth. Now the new midwife would shoulder the major responsibility, while her teacher offered her aid and counsel where needed. This system brought an abundance of tradition and consummate skill to the birthing bed. It was a long-standing and noble profession of women.

From the sunset review of the 1982 law came the 1984 midwifery statute. This law currently eliminates any further training or promotion of lay midwifery in the state of Florida. Those midwives with license in hand or women who enrolled in one of the two midwifery schools established since 1982 for their training toward licensing were exempted from this order. This places the number of potential and practicing midwives in Florida at thirty. The physicians won a decisive victory, allowing the thirty women to continue as a "compromise." And hospitals are incorporating birthing rooms and centers to adapt in some way to the home-birth trend. Freestanding birth centers, administered by nurse-midwives and lay midwives with sympathetic doctors serving as backup, are also making bids for respectability. Meanwhile, the few remaining black midwives of the rural South are taking their rich tradition with them to their graves.

> The gift. Now, if you got the gift . . . Mm-mmm, well, I'll tell you what, I delivered—I know you can't remember; it's before your time. You heard of the blackouts, when they wouldn't let you have lights in the house at night. I don't know if you heard about that. They was afraid to have lights in the house. And I delivered a baby during that without a light. I just felt my way. You got a guide; the Lord is with you, and you have a guide. You have somebody to teach you. . . . I thank the Lord; every time I turn around, I'm thankful. He's been too good to me.[27]

Chapter Four

A Rebirth of
American Midwifery

I remember my first interview; it was with a black midwife in northern Florida. The meeting was arranged by a young woman whose first child had been delivered by the midwife years before. We took the long drive out to the country, and from memory my friend found her way back to the place where she had undergone the metamorphosis of woman into mother. As we entered the small, neat home, family members cleared the room, making way for my first sight of her. She was large and dark and dignified, and she sat in a vinyl recliner across from a huge color television. On the opposite wall from where I sat hung a gallery of small faces, each vying for her attention. She remained seated as we were introduced and looked every inch the noblewoman I had expected. By this time, feeling quite impressionable, I braced myself as one who has been granted an audience with some noted sage. She, on the other hand, was baffled at my visit, assuming that I had come for only one of two reasons: I was seeking to apprentice or in need of a delivery. When I told her I had never had a child and was not then pregnant, she winked at my companion and said, "I guess we're gonna have to break her in."

Between them the women passed a message, communicated in winks and laughter; having once shared a childbirth together, only they could fully appreciate its meaning. The implication was that I, under their tutelage, could also be initiated into this experience with them. This attitude toward childbirth was different from what I was used to. It embraced an air of confidence and power that seemed rooted in an esoteric knowledge that was potentially open to me. *They,* the initiates, would break me, the novitiate, in. And then they winked and laughed. The women offered to conduct me on the journey to my new status, and it was childbirth—not sex or marriage or age or education—that would make me one with them. They were possessors of an ancient prerogative that would aid in my transformation. And they winked and laughed. Once completing my rite of passage, I would be winking with them. There must be a history behind their self-assured grins—a long line of winkers.

> I remember it distinctly with my first child, which was thirteen and a half years ago. And it was almost indescribable; it was just a real feeling of kinship with all women everywhere, pretty much. You know, just knowing that women since the beginning of time had been doing that and that that's why we were all here, was very reassuring. It was like almost an initiation rite or something. I guess in a primitive sense, that's what it was. I didn't think of it that way at the time, but later on processing the experience I came to think of it that way. And I would think that women giving birth with other women present would feel a real bond with those women. I didn't have that experience because I had a male obstetrician and the nurses in the hospital who were really pretty faceless to me. They all had masks on and we didn't have any kind of relationship. But at the same time I still felt that. So I would think that it would just be even *more* so with women who are really connected with each other.[1]

Grounded in a healthy scientific outlook and reared by technology, the young, white, and middle class went home and did the unthinkable: they invited the midwife back to deliver their babies the old-fashioned way. In comparing the interviews of the old women with those of the young, I noticed a contrast of tones.[2] The young women looked with wonder and amazement upon aspects of their births for which the old women displayed little excitement. While the older women took a lot for granted, the young mothers, all good feminists, found in their women-attended births a power their ideologies had somehow missed. The young mothers spoke of a deeper-felt female camaraderie that crossed all cultural borders and spanned generations of time. They even extended this feeling to their mothers and grandmothers, from whom they had felt estranged. A new meaning and respect for "woman's intuition" was awakened in those who felt they would have not endured the transition stage without the strength in their midwives' eyes. And each raved proudly of a strong body and the undaunted force with which it worked to deliver the child—flexing muscles like an amateur weight lifter.

I asked the older women about the spiritual aspects of birth, whether there was something cosmic about it. Was there not something electric going on among women at a birth? While the young women eagerly devoured these questions, the old women responded with blank stares. My rephrasings only elicited answers that had little to do with the questions, and wisely, I took this as a sign. The questions were not questions but ideological statements in search of confirmation. They reflected a one- or two-generation time warp in which birth as a source of female power had lain dormant, and having rediscovered it as such, we (my generation and I) were excited about its implications for our view of women as strong and powerful—something the older women had just assumed. The young mothers did not have this luxury. Their own mothers were asking them what birth was like. Modern medical practice had eclipsed at least two generations of women's shared experiences in childbirth, and a little excitement here and there at its resurrection was to be expected.

Middle-class midwifery is a movement to take back this right of childbirth. It is replete with feminist ideology, reacting to fifty years of stolen goods. Birthing fads such as underwater childbirth, champagne breakfasts, and videotaped labors are not the only reasons that the new midwifery will never be the old midwifery. The latter evolved organically from a culture, while the former is a self-conscious acculturation. The home-birth movement is sometimes hard put to forsake altogether its middle-class attachments to legal, scientific, and academic institutions. And the new midwifery's pursuit of legal recognition through state licensure perpetuates the old model of state control. Compromise with the state has led to the state's successful attainment of a long-awaited goal: the replacement of the traditional lay midwife with the modern nurse-midwife. And in so doing, the state permanently altered a cultural tradition, forcibly ended a respected woman's trade, and systematically distorted an important segment of women's history—in particular, the history of Northern ethnic and Southern black women.

Perhaps the only injustice that can be corrected now is this one of history. The study of the old midwife model offers a rare piece of history in which women are defined on their own terms and in which working-class women are presented in leadership roles. This is a departure from a traditional history that assumes man to be the measure of significance and poses questions about women's history within that context. This greatly restricts women's history to those women who achieved notoriety within, or significantly reacted against, the patriarchy. Historically recognizing only women who contributed to male history is a negative approach to women's history.[3] Midwifery offers a unique look at women's culture outside the realm of men, one that evolved from and was framed by the needs of women. Midwifery is an institution that virtually precedes male culture, as opposed to reacting to it; so its history is a uniquely positive one. "That's all was going with no doctors, 'cause they never come in them days. Nothin' but midwives. And they just cut off all those midwives. . . . But I believe they should go back and *get* those midwives."[4]

The Interviews

Interview with Augusta Wilson, August 6, 1981

Mrs. Wilson, a black midwife, practiced in a growing
north-Florida town, where she estimates to have delivered five hundred babies. She had her license taken
away, without a hearing, when a baby died at a birth
she was attending. She claims the family, who were
members of the Holiness Church, created such a scene
of religious fervor that the young woman in labor became frightened and her contractions stopped. Against
the advice of Mrs. Wilson, the family delayed in transporting the woman to the hospital, and the baby died.

When was your last delivery?

In 1965.

You don't deliver as a favor to close friends when asked?

Oh, yes. I do that if somebody comes asks me to help 'em out. The doctors's experimentin' on the midwives. They happen to be takin' care of 'em, but a doctor ain't never had no baby. A man ain't never had no baby. He don't know how . . .

They are trying hard to phase the midwives out.

Well, I know. That's what happened here in L—— County. We had a doctor that was with the clinic, and he just didn't like midwives. Well, I ain't ashamed to say who—Dr. A—— was one. He just despised midwives. He told me he "hated the damn midwives." And there's a lot of young women—a lot of people—who can't *afford* to go to the hospital. And the midwives, you see, the midwives took care of the women. The doctor doesn't care. All they want is they money. And we always had to visit the mother the whole time during her pregnancy and help her get ready for her delivery.

Now, they had prenatal care under the doctor, you know. The doctor had to check 'em, but we had to go and help 'em get the baby—show 'em how to sew. Like a young mother who never had a baby, she didn't know how to sew. So then you had to show her how to prepare for her delivery. We would show her how to make clothes and show her how to get herself ready—her sanitary pieces, if she couldn't buy Kotex. Well, we would get cloths; she'd wash and wring them, roll them in the shape of a napkin, fold 'em, wrap 'em in brown paper and put 'em in the oven; bake them thirty to forty minutes and pack them in a box. We would get the gowns ready, put them in a box, suitcase, whatever they had that was convenient. We would put her there. Well, to take care of the baby—even the baby, we would put bands on the baby. Now they don't put anything, and here the baby with a navel that long. We put bands on the baby to take care of the baby's navel until it come off. 'Cause, you see, the mother couldn't diaper or handle on it or nothing, and upsettin' the navel where most of the babies get infected, they end up with navels that long. And the doctors will tell you, "Oh, well, you can't do nothing about that big navel." That's not true. That's not true. And I have proof.

How many babies have you delivered?

About five hundred.

Did you ever use forceps?

Well, we never used 'em. Just used our hands. Never allowed us to use them.

Do you think they're necessary?

I don't think so.

How about cutting?

No, we never cut the woman. I had one or two to tear. 'Cause when the head presents down in the mouth of the pelvis, I always got a real hot cloth and press right down low down against it, and that helped the mother to stretch, to relax.

Some midwives say they bring their Bibles to a birth. Did you?

No, I never did. Because I found that you didn't want to make them sad. You have to keep their minds off the baby. So I always joked, cut the fool with 'em. Reading the Bible—it's always making 'em think about they gonna die or something like that. We always joked with 'em—tried to make 'em forget the pains. Oh, I heard that, but I found that didn't work. Now if *they* wanted to do it, that was *them.* I'd joke around and cut the fool with 'em and tease 'em and go on. And after a while, they get to laughing and talking and relax theyselves. And sometimes, first thing, here the baby, and then some don't think about the pains or what they was going through.

Do you think the story of Eve in the Bible concentrates a lot on the pain of birth and its sinful nature?

Oh, I mean, the ones that just want to believe in it or want to go along with it—but just. . . . Well, now *listen,* I *have* religion. I'm a religious person. I believe in God. I have a *strong* faith; I have a *strong* belief in God. And I believe I know what God will do, but *still,* there's a way—there's so many places you can use God. And this mother—a woman having a baby—she thinks about God, but they is more—some of 'em has *never* had a baby. They afraid, and when you go to readin' the Bible and prayin' with 'em, you gets them nervous. You get 'em all [so] they think they in danger. And having a baby—if they do—if blood pressure is down, the kidneys is alright, it's no danger. It's no emergency case, see? So I found out that the more you tease 'em, joke, and carry on with 'em, the better they get along. I had one woman, she had a baby, and she was, oh, at least her family was, Holiness. And they just started to jumpin' up and shoutin' and carryin' on in the room where the woman were. And "thank God and holy come on Jesus!" They got her so nervous, the pains cut off. She couldn't get no contractions. She just give up. The baby died. Because, you see, it caught him right across his neck when her pains cut off. And before he could get her to the hospital, the baby died. She'd choked him to death.

Why didn't you send the relatives out of the room?

They wouldn't go *out.* They was so holy and sanctified and well satisfied.

What do you think of having fathers in the room at birth?

I think if a woman wants her husband in there, there's nothin' wrong with it. Course, I never wanted *mine* in there, but I have had so many mothers wanted their husbands. 'Cause [with] some of 'em, wasn't nobody there but the father *and* I. I had to have him to help 'cause some mothers was just a little bit unruly. And I had to have his help. So me and fathers have delivered a *lot* of babies. [Laughter.] They's a help. Then a lot of mothers want their husbands. They *call* for him. So since *they* want him, I call him in.

How many children did you have?

Seven.

Another midwife delivered you?

Yeah.

Why are women going back to midwives?

Why? Because it's cheaper. And it's better. 'Cause when a woman have a baby at home, she have more privileges. See, she can walk. Like a pain hit her, she can get up and walk around that chair, or she can walk around. A woman can move around during her labor. But you see, in the hospital, no quicker than you get there they put you in that bed and let you *stay* there by yourselves. They going on about their business, or there the nurse over there with her feet in the chair reading. The doctor home laid up with his legs crossed reading a book. And there *you* in the room by yourself. But now you're home, the midwife is sitting there. *You* have changed your bed; it's all fixed, and *you* have the chance to walk around. And the *only* time you're supposed to confine a mother to the bed is when her membrane erupts. And then when *that* happens, then you supposed to confine her to the bed because it's nothin' to take care of the baby's head. And the baby's head falls right down in the mouth of the [pelvis]. See, you close it and mash his head up, crush his head. But then you confine her to the bed. But until that happens, she can move around.

*   *   *   *   *

Well, you see [in the hospital], they don't pay 'em no mind, 'cause I remember my daughter-in-law was in the hospital. She hadn't had a baby in twelve years. She called me that morning at three o'clock and told me she was in labor.

Didn't she want you to deliver it?

No, she *had* to go to the hospital. And so I asked her how close was the pains. And she told me. So I said, "Well, alright, just go on back and lie down till it be about thirty minutes apart." I say, "But if it come down so she see it"—and I said then it would be about thirty minutes apart. I said, "Unless you start seeing signs of her membrane broke, and then you take her to the hospital." So then her husband called me and told me they were start to seeing signs. So I said, "Well, take her on in." He take her to the hospital three o'clock that morning. It her first baby [and] she ain't supposed to stay in labor no longer than twenty-four hours. She in there eighteen hours. And she was in labor from three o'clock that morning until ten o'clock that night. It was four o'clock then before he called me and come got me and take me up to the hospital. And when I went to the hospital, she was still laying in the bed, still having pains. So the nurse say, "She isn't ready yet." So I was sitting there. I went on in there, and there's Aileen. I said to her, "Does the nurse know your membrane had erupt?" She said, "No, I don't think—*I think she do!*" That's what she said. And the pains then were about four minutes apart. And she was having *hard* pains. And for every pain she had, she kinda shook like that. So then I went and said, "Did you know?" I says, "Where's the doctor?" The nurse say, "He's home." I said, "Well, I want to *talk* to him. *You* call him and tell him to come to the hospital. I want to *talk* with him." Well, they think they know it all. I say, "Well, I'll tell you one thing, her membrane is erupted." And I said, "He's going to be delivering a *dead* baby instead of a *live* baby if he don't get here and do something about this woman. She ain't got no business being in labor this long." I said, "If she can't have it, he should have done something." I say, "Now—" That time she jumped up there and then run. She say, "Goodness! We got to—we got to call the doctor." So she run in there. She was about to try to push the bed through the window for the door. [Laughter.] Finally, she got her out and take her on down to the operating room. See, he was almost dead. He weighed ten pounds, but they had to put him in the incubator. He was almost—he was almost dead.

How old was she when she had the baby?

Mm-mmm. Oh, she was about thirty.

Why couldn't she have the baby? Was it too large?

Yeah, she couldn't have a baby that large. A smaller baby that didn't weigh but five pounds, the doctor had to take *that* one. And he knew it all the time. And he should have took the baby. He knowed he was a large baby. She would have no way in the world give birth to him. And he *knew* it.

Did you ever deliver any of your grandchildren?

Yeah. It's just like anybody else's.

Can you remember an unusual birth out of those five hundred?

Yeah, I had one—his buttocks come first. And then I had one the knee come first.

Even that mother didn't tear?

I didn't even try to deliver. When I found [out] I rushed her down to the hospital. You see, I never let my mothers suffer. Because, see, when I found that one couldn't have a baby, I didn't want that she would suffer. I just called the doctor.

How many other mothers did you take to the hospital?

Oh, about ten.

Ten out of five hundred is pretty good.

Well, I would say I had pretty good luck. I think about two, three stillbirths.

How about breast-feeding?

I always encourage all my mothers, the ones that wanted to—and a lot of 'em didn't want to. But I encouraged them and they did. At least, I tell 'em, they should nurse their babies a month; and I had to work with that. Mother's milk *always* better for a baby! And then it makes you closer to your baby when you nurse your baby. You are closer to your baby. You loves it. You learns to care for it. And then the child is closer to *you*. I think that's a lot of why so many mothers and children are so far apart today. Because *all* of my children—I breast-fed every *one* of 'em. And all of my children, they're real close. You're always closer to them. You *feels* closer to them. Even to my daughter-in-law here. She went to the hospital for her first child; she got a little boy. He's five now. And she said she wasn't gonna nurse him. I said, "You're gonna nurse him." I said, "Now, don't think nothing else. Because you want your child to *love* you." And I said, "You want to be close to your family, then nurse him." So she did, and the doctor tried to talk her out of it. And she still told me she was gonna breast-feed it. He went and told her he would give her a shot to dry up her milk so she wouldn't. So I told her, "Tell him don't give you no shot. You want to use your breast. Tell him . . ." So she did. She nursed it, and she tells me, "I'm *so* glad you encouraged me to nurse my baby, 'cause I feel so close to her [*sic*] by nursing." And she say, "If I hadn't a nursed him, I wouldn't have felt this close." But I think any mother should nurse her baby two or three months. And I don't tell 'em not to give 'em a bottle. 'Cause sometimes you are busy. So if you're busy, you always give 'em the bottle. Just like we have to leave 'em. You don't have to knock your brains out gettin' back home to feed it. Then you give 'em a bottle. That's what I always did, and that's what I did for her. She nursed him, and then she would give him the bottle when she was away. And when you get ready to wean 'em, you just stop nursing 'em. You give 'em the bottle. Listen, I had one of mine—my baby—he stopped nursin' on his own, but all the rest of 'em had to be [weaned]. They won't give it up. One of 'em was big. He would go catch me and push me down in the chair. [Laughter.] He'd get in front of me, you know. And I'd back right back to a chair, and he would kinda push me. I would let him push me, and I would sit down in a chair. Then he would sit up in my lap. He would crawl in my lap, and I'd nurse him, and then he'd go to sleep. So they want to nurse—they'll nurse till they're ten years old if you don't wean them.

What do you have to say on illegitimate children?

They all *children* to me. I mean, to me they aren't different from any children. 'Cause now all *my* children had the same daddy. I stayed there until I knew I was through having children 'cause I didn't want no mixed children. 'Cause it makes the meanest children. I don't care if you quit your husband and marry again and have children for another man, they still a mean set of children. I prayed and asked God to let me live till my baby get grown, till they could take care of themselves. 'Cause I didn't want—see, I devoted all my time to my children. My husband and I separated when my children was small. The oldest one was just fifteen. So then I had to raise all of them, and I raised my six, and two or three of somebody else's.

> *Interview with Evelyn Reynolds, January–*
> *February 1983*
>
> Georgia Reynolds, now deceased, was a black urban
> midwife in Florida. She operated a thriving maternity
> home in the fifties and sixties. As her clientele dimin-
> ished over the years, she opened a senior citizens' home.
> Her daughter, Evelyn, the source for this interview, is
> now the director of that home. Members of her com-
> munity referred to the respected midwife as "Mother
> Reynolds."

I tried to figure out while you were gone how long ago she [Mother] started. From what I can figure, she must have started in that field of work either the late thirties or early forties, because I was figuring my daughter's birth. See, she was the last baby she delivered, and Kathy's twenty-four years old.

She delivered your baby?

Uh-huh. That was the *last* one.

What's it like having your mom deliver your baby for you?

Ahhh! I'll tell you what it was like. Ignoring me completely.

What?

Ignoring me completely. Well, the reason why I say that is because at that time she had the home, and I started going into light labor like about five something in the morning. And she told me, "Oh, just go back to bed. You'll be alright." It was my first baby, you know? [Laughter.] She'd told so many that, and to me it was just, "Hey, what is she talkin' about?" I'd seen so many women *have* babies and everything because I was right there in the home where I could watch her work, but all of a sudden it's my time, and it seems a little serious to me to say, "Go back to bed." So sure enough, I stayed up. I went and washed my car, I cleaned up my room . . .

You washed your car?

Mm-hmm. I did some of everything that day, and finally, I guess about twelve-thirty or one o'clock, the pains just got unbearable. So she carried me to the delivery room and got me all ready. And when I looked, she was outdoors doin' her laundry. I said, "Now, what is this!" You know? I'm gettin' real worried. She kept running in the house asking, "Well, how you doin'?" I say, "I'm doin' *terrible!*" "Well, now," she said, "I'm tellin' you now, you better get ready to uncross your legs; you can't have a baby with your legs crossed." And so finally she got downright busy with me 'cause the pains were so close to coming, and Kathy was born like about four forty-five in the afternoon. She waited many, many years to tell me why she stayed out of the room. I said, "Well, why is it? You used to hang around with everybody else and fan 'em and, you know, put cool pads on their face and rub their hands and rub their hips, so why you ignorin' me?" She says, "Well, with you, you were my daughter, and I hated to see you bear the pain. So I tried to time you by coming in and out checking on you." Sure enough, she was there when she was born, but it had me worried. [Laughter.] She had delivered babies throughout the family. Her brothers' wives' children, children's babies, and their wives' babies. But with me, I was pretty close, being an only daughter. So that's the last one she delivered.

Tell me about the delivery you made at age thirteen.

Well, I'll tell you how that came about. When she first opened a home, there was still some people who still wanted to have their babies at home. They would come over, the husband and wife, and look over the maternity home, but they still wanted to be home. And I think maybe not so much wanting to be home, they feared they didn't have anyone to look after the young ones that were home. My mother delivered sometimes as many as eight babies for one woman, and those babies were just like stair steps; they were havin' 'em every eighty days. That's the way it looked to me. Every time you turn around, the same woman was right back, ready to have a baby. So, many a time she would accommodate them by still goin' into the home to deliver the babies. This particular time, she had gone to check on a lady, and this lady, she came in—her husband brought her in like about eleven o'clock in the morning. I was at home, and this woman was rarin' to go. And I says, "Well, my God, Momma's not here." I didn't panic. I had seen her do it *so* many times. I just went right on in and got that paper tray and had him to put her little buttocks on that tray, scrubbed my hands, scrubbed her up and everything—I did this! I had seen my momma do it so many times. We were raised around this. So the baby just [slaps hands together] bob, just like that, here she comes, the little girl. After the baby was born, well, I knew better than to try to cut the umbilical cord, although I knew how to do it just as good. I'd seen my mother take the sterilized tape, tie it off, cut it, and how many inches to do it from the navel, but I wouldn't take a chance on *this*. I wrapped the baby up, made it very comfortable, 'cause she came here yellin'; there was no slappin' on the back. She just came here like, "Well, God, I'm glad to be here." The mother was very thrilled to see her here because evidently she'd been in a lot of pain, and the husband didn't think nothing of it. Then the baby started cryin'. "Well, you little rascal you," I said. "Evidently you want to eat." And I knew what my mother's philosophy was on that: always sterile sugar-water—sterilized bottle, nipple, water and everything. I gave her about an ounce of sterilized water, and she drank. As my mother came, she was laying down in between her mother's legs just as comfortable and sound asleep.

How long did she stay like that?

Stayed like that for approximately about an hour before Mother came.

And that's okay for an hour?

Mm-hmm. For an hour, it didn't matter.

How come she didn't breast-feed?

Well, I don't know whether she wanted to—I wouldn't have even thought about breast-feeding 'cause, see, I would have had to detach the umbilical cord to keep the strain off. So, I wouldn't even go into that, no way. But I wasn't afraid; I wasn't shaky or anything, because I had seen her deliver so many babies.

You didn't want to follow in that line of work?

Well, my mother always wanted me to go into that field of work. As a matter of fact, she wanted me to be a nurse. And I never really wanted to be a nurse, but then after I started growing up, I started thinking how nice it would have been to be a midwifery person. But I sort of look back and could remember how badly she felt when they pushed her out of the field. And in my day of studies and coming up in school, I couldn't see where that would be a field *ever* again a person would perform in the home. I couldn't see that. So I went on to school and studied home economics instead. But it's a strange thing. This hit upon my mind maybe about three or four years ago. I said, "You know, that's what I should do." Because I started reading things about it. I said to myself, I wouldn't need that many hours of studying just to go back to school and brush up on some of the fields from the areas that I would have to have and go into it from a professional standpoint. It's a joyous way to make a living to see a new life come into the world. Because, like I said, even at twelve, it didn't bother me, not one bit! And of course, I was very private about what had happened even as a kid in school. You would have thought I would have gone to school saying, "Look! Guess what I did!" I was never that type of child. My mother always instilled in us to be adults even when we were just children. And thank God that particular time she had because the husband probably would have just been frantic. But I guess he could look at me and say, "Here's a thirteen year old just movin' just like the mother would have done." Yeah, yeah [laughter], he wasn't concerned at all; if so, he didn't say anything. And when my mother came, she said, "Look what we have here. Look what Evelyn did for us!" Of course, that child was named after me, and I'm real proud. I don't know where she is today, but she was named Evelyn after me. So that's the reason why I didn't go into it, but it has gone on my mind the past few years—that's the type of work that [I] could enjoy because, like my mother, I'm a public servant. I enjoy working and doing for people. She wasn't the kind who did it for money because there's a lot of 'em would say, "Okay, I'm going to charge you fifty dollars for the birth of this child." Nine days of care, even many days before the child was even born, she would talk with the mother-to-be, see how she's doin', are you gainin' weight, are you seein' the doctor, are you getting your blood checked. Mother always did this kind of stuff *way* before the baby was born. And she would check on 'em to see if there was any swelling of the ankles, anything like this. She always checked this first many, many months before this child was born. And I more or less felt, after I saw what happened to her, that there was no way for me to go into that field of work. She would come home, and she would say, "Well, it's gettin' to the place that all of my patients, when I send 'em up to the clinic, they're tellin' 'em to go to the hospital." And there was a nurse, her name was A——, who was notorious for it. My mother's feelings were very, very hurt about it because she had done many years of *good* work. I know my brother would know because he's a little bit older than me, but I stayed very close to her and her work, and I can't recall her losin' but one mother—*one* mother! And this was because of the doctor. I would say he was assisting in the case. Maybe not—he didn't bring it on; maybe the mother didn't get the health care that she should have gotten. It could have been any number of reasons, but she ended up in labor, and my mother kept telling him, "Doctor, this is going to be a breech birth." And, of course, the lady was way up in age and hadn't had a child in like twelve years. And my mother knew it was going to be a difficult case, and she kept sayin', "This woman needs to go to the hospital." Of course, the husband insisted that he wanted this child delivered in the maternity home. So when she got really into it, when my mother knew of this problem, she called the doctor in on the case. He let the lady wear herself out for an entire night, and my mother kept sayin', "She's gotta go to the hospital." But I guess, bein' the doctor, he was gonna have the final say. So they finally did end up carryin' this lady to the hospital, and my mother used to *often* talk about it—what a brutal birth it was. She used to tell us how this doctor—she was allowed to go into the operating room—how this doctor literally pulled this baby out piece by piece, and before day that morning, that mother actually did die.

After that delivery you did, did you feel any pressure from anyone to go into midwifery?

Yes, quite a few people in the community used to always say, "Well, you just go ahead and be a midwife just like your mother." But by the time I got ready to go to school, she had had such a hard time with it that I knew that that was no field for me to go into. And since then, I've often thought about it, but here recently it's just getting to the point now where women are ready to say, "Hey, I want to have the *right* to have my baby at home." They're actually standing up for that right, and I feel like they deserve that right as long as there's someone there who is experienced, who knows what she's doin'—or he—and if they find out there's difficulties, they shouldn't be selfish about it; they should get that person to a medical facility immediately.

Why did they try to push you to be a midwife?

I think maybe the long years of service that my mother gave, and she was so dedicated about it and loved it so much. This wasn't a fictitious type thing. People could see that. I also assisted her in many, many ways as a child growing up. For an example, when she did come to set up her own business at home, I did everything from helping her to put people to bed, roll 'em out on the stretcher (her homemade stretcher—she didn't buy one; she built it herself) to helping her to change ladies in the evening to sitting there entertaining the family members as they would come in directly to where the mother was and bring the baby out for them to see—this type of thing. So it was something that I had started at early childhood just helping her. I'll never forget this: "You always wait on a patient with a *smile!*" she would always say. And if for some reason I'd come in from school and maybe I want to go to majorette practice instead of coming home and help her, you know, this thing happens when you're a teenager. You see other things you want to do. If I got a little bit salty about it, and I didn't want to go, you know what she would tell me? "Get that smile on your face before you go into the ward." She called it the ward, and I always had to carry that smile. So, I guess the people, even if some days I didn't *want* to be there, it looked as though I was happy, and a lot of times I was. It's just some evenings I wanted to go be a majorette worse than going home to help her. But I think this is what brought that about: people seeing me in the field of work with her. I didn't do any of the deliveries other than the one that I did when she wasn't at home. But I did a lot of work, like I did a lot of birth certificates. My mother wasn't a highly educated woman, and as I grew up, I learned how to do the insurance forms for her; I did the birth certificates for her; I did most of the bookkeeping for her. I was just really right—her partner, so to speak. I guess this is what brought people around to thinking that it would be a good field of work for me, too.

But not your brothers. It wouldn't be good for them? Did they help as much?

The biggest thing that my oldest brother often used to get caught in was picking ups. And by pickin' up, I mean that maybe someone's ready to come into the home to have a baby, but there's no car in the home, no transportation, and he has had to go as far as fourteen miles out of T—— into the country, the rural areas, and pick ladies up. I remember one day my mother sent him out to W—— to pick up a lady. If he were here, he could tell you the same thing. He thought this lady was going to have this baby on that backseat any minute. And he said, "I was scared; I was just scared to death." He said, "Mama, I'm just *not* going to pick up another lady. There is no way!" He says, "I'm not going to do it ever again!" And he never did. She never forced him to go because being a young man, I guess she could see that that was getting on his nerves. He was about sixteen or seventeen years old then, going out to pick up a female having a baby! But many a time, the work called for this. Either they wanted to stay home or they would come into the home with no transportation or no one to stay with the younger children. So it was always a problem, and mother was the type of person that just tried to work *with* the problem and work *with* the client all at the same time regardless what the problem was. So many a time, in her eagerness to do this, it more or less just took the whole *family* to help do it, whatever it was. You just did it, and that was it.

What did your father do?

My father was a railroad man, retired after about thirty-some years with the Seaboard Coastline Railroad. Mm-hmm. And he mostly worked at night; so that worked out convenient for them. Yeah, because most babies, it seems, for some reason, are born at night, and my father would be gone to work; so, that helped my mother a lot, too.

Talk about how she felt when she closed her maternity home.

She began to sense that something was going on. At first, she thought it was a good thing that she could go up to the clinic and meet her mothers up there. And a lot of times, she didn't meet her mothers up there; she would go and pick up four and five women who didn't have transportation, carry them to meet the maternity clinic, and help them to weigh them, working *with* the staff. This is the type of thing that she *thought* was a betterment for all concerned. But as it worked out, she found out a lot of her clients—clients she had delivered four and five babies for—were beginning to tell her, "Well, Mis' Reynolds, Mis' A—— is telling me I need to go to the hospital." And Mother says, "Well, let me get on the phone and talk with her and see if there's any complications setting in. Because if there were, well, it was okay. If they feel like they found somethin' wrong with your blood or something wrong with your urinary system or something, then you *need* to go." But there wouldn't be anything wrong with them. She would actually check it out. And what happened, they would attend this clinic, and eventually, after attending so many times—I think they went like once a month or once every two weeks—they would give them a card stating that they were alright for midwifery delivery and more or less okay from the clinic. And all of a sudden Mama wasn't getting any cards. Of course, during this same time she started listening to what some of the clients were saying. She would also talk with Mrs. Barton [another midwife in town] about it. And the two started just feeling the pinch. At first Mrs. Barton was saying that she wasn't having any problems. And I think, for a while, that brought on a little rivalry between Mrs. Barton and Mama. But pretty soon, even Mrs. Barton found it out. I'm sure—and she would probably end up telling you this—that pretty soon everybody ends up being shuttled out to the hospital. So Mother found out there was nothing that she could do about it. You can't beat the system when you got the doctors out there saying do this, and then you got the nurses out there saying do this. No one is giving you any feedback as to *why* it's happening, but you see it happening. It got to the place that Mother's ward was just catching dust, and I seen the time the calendar was just lined *up* with babies being born. She had two delivery rooms, as I said, and those delivery rooms were hot; she kept them busy from one to the other having a baby and taking care of them, seeing about them, and their food, 'cause she took care of the whole bit. They even had their food while they were there, and she did their laundry, everything! Even to the point that sometimes, if they didn't have transportation, *she* carried them home with the husband's help. She just got to the place where she just sat there and she looked at her equipment—no deliveries, no one coming. And she got, well, I would say, at first, she got a little angry about it. This type of thing, someone killing your career, is just like killing some member of the family that's real close. At first, she began to wonder. You ask yourself questions, "Well, what have *I* done wrong?" You look back, and you say, "I've delivered maybe thirty or forty babies a month, on the average, for years. And I've only lost one mother, and that mother was lost in a hospital with the doctor attending." And you haven't had that many stillbirths, and you begin to wonder, "Well, what in the world am I doing wrong?" Then after a while, you start listening to your clients say, "Well, they want me to go to the hospital." You checked into that and found out that there's nothing physically *wrong* with this lady; why can't she still come into the home to have the baby? No one is giving any answers on it. So you just pretty soon feel whipped. And her equipment got whipped, and *she* got whipped. She just sat there and looked at her home, which was always done up in the prettiest white sheets that you want to lay your eyes on. She even *ironed* her mothers' sheets. They didn't have that much wash and wear back in those days. Mother never put a rough, dry cotton sheet on a lady's bed; they were *pressed;* pillowcases were starched! This is the kind of home that she ran. She just kept sittin' there lookin' at her equipment collect dust, and she'd go by and make the beds up, just hopin' things would get better. And they didn't ever get any better, to the point that she felt, "Well, I may as well just go into some other field of work." And that's when she decided in 1957—the fall of 1957—to go into setting up a home for senior citizens. And she went on to do that for another seventeen years before she passed.

Then the year that the home closed was 1957.

I would say it closed before then: in the early fifties. She couldn't *believe* what was going on, and she just kept sitting there hoping for the best that never came.

When did the home open?

I must have been about fifteen or sixteen years old at the time when it opened because we were young teenagers, and she didn't want us to be home alone. That was her reason for setting up the clinic at home. She didn't want to be away from home. She wanted to be able to peep in on the family as well as to do her work. There were two brothers, and I was the only girl in the home.

What year was it?

That's what I'm tryin' to figure out. Now, I was born in 1934, and I would say *definitely* she was at home doing deliveries by the time I was about fourteen years old. So, about the early fifties was when she started that home. About the late forties and early fifties is when she built that home. And building that home, she started a career for another member of her family. She told my uncle, "I gotta have a building." She says, "I know just how I want it built." And he says, "What do you mean you're goin' to have a building?" "Well, I'm going to bring my work home." And my father said, "Well, you must be crazy. You're out of your mind talkin' about building a maternity home." [Laughter.] And she just got out there, and she figured out how long a bed was and how wide a bed was and how many feet and inches it would take up. She knew how many she wanted to have on each side of the wall. She must have had about a ten- or twelve-feet span. She wanted it large enough to be able to wheel 'em from the delivery room into their bed area. And it was an open ward type thing with windows on each side, and eventually she put an air conditioning system in and everything. And my uncle, who was also a person who did *not* finish school, but was a person who was always very skillful, had never laid any block in his life. She said, "But you can do it. I'm going to show you how to do it." Now, she had never laid any either. So he ended up building that place at the corner of B—— and 22nd on a very busy street in T——. And *so* many people passed; they saw his work, they liked his work. He didn't know what he was doin', but he started a career that lasted another thirty-some years in the building trade. Mm-hmm.

Did you say that your mother felt betrayed?

Yes, she did. She felt betrayed by the state. She knew that the state was behind it. But I think she felt, "Well, here they are. They've got more education than I have, they have more trainin' than I have, they're sayin' that this is the way it should be done. They're not tellin' me why. This is just it!"

But she was never illegal.

No, no. She always had her license, kept it current. Her place was inspected all the time.

Tell me about those inspections.

One of the nurses or someone would come by and look at it, and would say, "Well, everything looks real nice and sanitary." Because she had to keep everything sanitary, from the kitchen where she prepared the food to right down to where they lived, and both the babies' rooms—'cause she had rooms that the babies stayed in; they didn't stay with the mother until feeding time. Then she would bring—just about like they do in a hospital now—she would bring the babies out.

Other than that, she just kept a [vigilant] watch over the babies, *and* over the mothers, day and night. That was her job. And they always told her everything looked real nice. Like I said, I think she just got tired of waiting and knew that she couldn't beat the system. So she just gave up.

Someone has told me that they would run a series of spot inspections on some clinics in an effort to close them down.

We never had that type of inspection. No, [they] just stopped referring people and stopped saying that you could go to the home.

So they just stopped issuing those little cards.

That's right, those little cards—blue and green. Some of 'em were green and some of 'em were blue. I imagine I probably still have some of those cards. They just stopped givin' 'em the cards to come. Now, keep it in mind, most of these people didn't have the money to go to a private doctor, so naturally they were *glad* to go to a clinic. They didn't have to pay this money for this prenatal care. And quite naturally, if the nurse and the doctor say, "Well, Mrs. Jones, you're to go to the hospital and have your baby," they didn't question it. And some of them *did* question it now.

How could they afford it?

That's what *I* can't understand. How did they do this?

They were probably doing it with—

Medicaid? Aren't they? Well, they didn't have medicaid during that time.

Well, now they're doing it. They say only certain practitioners are eligible, and the midwife isn't one of them. That's how they're doing it in G—— County.

Well, see, back in the early forties and fifties, there was no such thing as that kind of help to have a baby. I don't know how they influenced those ladies to go to the hospital. And they probably had to *pay.* I don't know how they managed to do it. I don't think they did it through scare tactics. I don't think they did it that way. They might have just gained their confidence in attending the clinic.

Do you remember any of those women? They must have been good friends of your mother, coming to her and feeling apologetic, feeling bad.

Yes, they sure did! A lot of 'em. As a matter of fact, even down to the day we buried her, we received calls from everywhere. People came from everywhere. And the one thing they wanted to talk about was her work as a midwife, about what a good job she had done. As a matter of fact, I was talking to a lady—it happened no more than three or four weeks ago—and she was telling me that she had carried her son to the funeral home to [view] the remains, and at that time, he was about twenty-some years old. He didn't even *know* my mother. My mother had delivered him, and he wanted to see this person who had brought him into the world. And I said, "Well, my goodness, I never realized all that went on at funeral time." She'd gotten telegrams, phone calls, oh, my goodness, the people! And that was one of the things that so many of 'em wanted to talk about, was how many babies—Mother's got babies all over this United States, everywhere! And you know, it was a good thing for her, like she said, it was something that she wanted to do from early childhood. I'm just real happy that she was able to carry out a childhood dream. But the dream just, for some reason or another, could not fight red tape, couldn't fight the system; this is happening now in a lot of fields of work, especially when you have the government now cutting in and helping out. The same thing is happening in my field of work that I'm in right now. I know that this is what is going on. Well, when you find out, you're certainly not going to try to buck the system. What are you gonna do when you got so many strong people out there saying, "Well, you gonna do it this way"? You just eventually kinda forget about it is what you do.

I have this idea about the destruction it does to cultural traditions: neighborhoods, community, black culture, etc.

Right, right, this is right. Mm-hmm. This is true.

And it kind of neutralizes everything.

Mm-hmm. That's the truth. Get to be like a "me, too" society. Everything's like "me, too!" You know, this is the [feeling]: it's like when they go out at U.S. Homes and look at their new homes, you leave away with that "me, too" feeling. "Me, too" America. Everybody looks alike; everything is alike. So this is the system that we live in, and for some reason, these things happen! *I* would be one of the first ones to say that if aboveboard care isn't given, then a person should not be in that field of work—any field, if you're workin' for people. It appears to me that if this was a strong fear during those years—there's a lot of people doing this type of work, and it appears to me there were shortcomings—that someone could have said, "Hey, let's shape these ladies up. Let's get 'em back to class." But that was never done. No one ever offered that type of assistance. It was just like, all of a sudden, "We don't need you any more, and we're not goin' to call you and tell you thanks for what you *have* done; we're not goin' to call you and tell you what you're doing wrong; we're not here to give you a hand to see what we can do to help you, either." It was just a thing that she felt completely numb about, I guess, and there was nothing she could do. But it really worried her; it really worried her. If she hadn't gone on into opening up a home for senior citizens, I don't know what would have happened to her. Because she was a person who was dedicated to humanity, working with mankind; that was her life! So thank God, someone needed her.

People at the health department really seem to just not know what happened. I'll ask, "Why did they close them?" They'll say, "Well, I don't know, really. Maybe it was high mortality rate."

Uh-uh. Now, I'll tell you what you've got to consider here. We're speaking about quite a few years back, and it could be, at the health department, there are not too many people that's in there working now who really, really understand what happened. They were probably somewhere in school, I guess, when all of this was going on 'cause we're talkin' about quite a few years back. I don't feel like the public ever really understood. So a lot of people don't know, but I'm thinkin' there's a lot of people at the health department that really wouldn't know.

So your mother never lost a baby.

Yes, she did. She had a couple stillborn; but Mother never had but a few stillborns, just a few. Most of her babies were born yellin' and kickin' and screamin'; most of 'em was. And the only mother [to die] that I knew of was the one with the breech birth. And [Mother] kept tellin' the doctor that she *knew* that it was gonna be a breech birth, and she needed to get the lady to the hospital, and finally, once he *did* carry her, she was just so worn out in the way that he went at the delivery—that thing haunted her for years. She used to always talk about how bad she felt that it had to happen that way.

What was her feeling about the medical profession in the beginning?

From the very beginning, the only thing that she had to do was to take so many hours training under a medical doctor. It was just okay, and nobody was makin' a big deal of it, only that she had to deliver so many babies—I have forgotten how many—but she had to go on actual deliveries before they could certify her as a midwife. She had a certificate from the state of Florida as having completed studies. And then later on, these nurses, I guess, wanted to further their studies, and they would more or less get 'em together, and they would have to go to the health department or someplace, and bring their bags in; they had to read so many chapters in a book, be able to interpret what they had read. They were able to practice, and the nurses assisted them with it at first. I don't know just what happened. All of a sudden they just wanted everybody to go to the hospital.

What was her standing in the black community that she lived in? Was she a church woman, respected . . .

I hate to use this word, but one way to describe her in the community was a God-sent love to the whole community—black and white. People loved her, admired her, respected her to the top. People thought there was nothing like her: Miss Reynolds, Miss Reynolds . . . If you were gonna have a baby, this is the lady you wanted to see. And some of 'em referred to her as Mother Reynolds because they felt like she had that motherly care and feeling for them. Even up to the day we buried her—even *now* I'm running into people. Sometime in my career as a teacher, I've been in a classroom, and kids will come up to me and say, "I knew your mother." "What do you mean, you knew my mother? You're too young." You know, [he's not] but twelve, thirteen years old. "Well, my mother knew your mother. She delivered me."

Tell me again the number of clients she averaged?

On the average, I would say at least forty-some babies per month or better. That's the way she averages the early years of her career. This is also one of the reasons she imagined having a place, a facility for them to come to. It was difficult to be on one case for two or three days, and you've got somebody else out there might need your services also. I believe this played heavily on her mind—as well as being home with us—that she needed a place, a facility to deliver her babies. You know, "Here I am, I'm permanent, and you can come in," this type of thing, because she was getting so many calls. She had so many clients. She kept a little card box, about like an index file-card [box, with information about] patients coming in to have babies.

Midwifery was one of those rare professions in which women could be leaders of a community. Do you want to say anything on that? Did you know any other midwives?

There was another lady we used to call Mother Catherine, who used to deliver babies—a real old lady. And there must have been at least four or five during the time. I think this way maybe Mother had caught on the idea of going more into it from some of the older ones. And maybe by the time she and Mrs. Barton got into it, some of them were beginning to taper off from the work. It was getting to be too strenuous for them, gettin' up all times of night, goin' out to deliver babies.

But she didn't apprentice under any of those older midwives?

No, no. Under a doctor. But you know, you have brought up something here that I am searching—I'm questioning—myself. If there was no real reason why they did it other than for money, that couldn't have been the reason, because a lot of these people were just poor people. They didn't have the money.

I don't know, that's what everyone seems to believe. It was more money according to most. It didn't seem to be a problem in places where there was no hospital, but when the first hospital was erected, the midwives seemed to follow a pattern of being phased out. I think also it's a certain scientific attitude we carry about things.

I think, yeah, could be. This is what I'm saying. I don't think anyone did it. Really, when I sit back and evaluate it, I think at that time they felt like, "Hey, this is the best place for a baby to be born, is in a hospital." I really believe that's what they felt. And in some cases, even with my mother, so far as that's concerned, maybe there were some shortcomings there that *I'm* not even aware of that made people feel like this is the best thing to do. I don't know; it's hard just to say. I would think that that's just a scientific feeling, a feeling that people had at that time that, "Well, all babies need to be born in the hospital because there may be complications." You just really don't know *what* they were thinking. But I have a feeling it wasn't so much as to maybe destroy midwifery as it was a strong feeling of helping the newborn and the mother-to-be by making sure that it was done under the safest and the most sanitary conditions. And this could have been rectified also *with* the midwifery field if someone had taken time to see it as being a type of cultural thing that they wanted to be maintained in this country.

Interview with Jenny Black, August 5, 1981

Mrs. Black is a sixty-year-old north-Florida black woman whose midwife had not only been employed by her mother but was present at all but one of her own births. After her midwife died, Mrs. Black took her last birth to the hospital.

How many children did you have at home?

Five.

Are they all still living?

No.

How many are still living?

Three.

You didn't lose the other two in childbirth?

I had two of 'em home. The last one I had was in the hospital.

What year was that?

That was in '62.

And why did you have that one in the hospital?

Well, because the lady that I was using had passed.

Tell me, how were they different?

I don't know if it was so much as *different.*

Were you awake?

Yes, I was always awake. I don't think there was too much a difference.

You don't prefer one over the other? If you were to have a baby now, would you have it at home?

Well, no, I would rather go to the hospital. And it was a little bit different because I think the doctor can kinda *help* you a little bit, seem like to me. I had one pain, and it really stopped [me, and] something he did, he kinda opened me up.

Did it take any longer?

No, it was quicker. Because by the time I got in the hospital, I had broke my water. I told them to call the doctor. They didn't. They says it wasn't time. She say, "Who the nurse?" I say, "You, but I'm the one deliverin' the baby." She *still* wouldn't call the doctor.

Why did she say she wouldn't?

'Cause she said it wasn't *time.* But my water broke in the bed. And you know, she picked up a towel, a big ol' bath towel, and rolled that thing and balled it up; she put it down here [points to her vagina] and got another one and crossed my legs. And I said, "Uh-uh, oh, no, you won't kill me like *this!*"

What did you think she was trying to do?

Keep the baby from coming, and the child was so near.

Why would she do that?

The doctor wasn't there, you know, and then I was in the bed.

She wanted you in the delivery room.

Oh, she was going on, "Blow out ja' mouth, blow out ja' mouth." The pain struck me so hard. I took my foot and shoved her over to that wall. [Laughter.] I wasn't gonna let her kill me and the child. By the time they got me in the delivery room and throwed me over there, that child's *head* came.

Was the doctor there?

No. And by the time he walked in, the child was almost all the way here. [The nurse] didn't even prep me. See, she waited so late, then she was goin' to prep me. I said, "Well, you ain't goin' to put no razor on me." And, whoa, them pains hit me, and I'm jumpin'. "You just have to be still." I said, "Nuh-uh!"

Did you get your way on that?

Yep. [Laughter.] I said, "You ain't gonna put that razor on me, and I mean it." I had a little ol' jar of deodorant that I got, and I was gonna let her have it. 'Cause I won't let her cut me with that razor.

You were going to spray her with the deodorant? You had to really fight her?

Because she didn't have any right. I kept telling her that it was time.

Was she helping you then with the baby as it was coming out? You said it was almost there.

No, she was trying to push it back! With a big towel, just like that, hollering, "Hold the legs, hold the legs!" Then she say, "You have a baby like a cat have kittens." I go, "Well, you must be the cat had the kittens." I told her from the time I got there to call the doctor. And the other lady say, "Is this your first child?" I said, "No." She said, "How many children do you have?" I said, "This is my fifth one." She said, "Don't you think she should know what she's talking about if she had five children?" I say to the nurse, "Call the doctor." She just said, "It's not time" [in mocking voice].

Was she a young nurse?

No, she was an old nurse. She say, "You gonna get an 'F' for the day." The doctor say, "How long has she . . ." "She just *got* here. She just got in the hospital." I says, "Doctor, I hadn't just got here." I say, "I've been here ever since a quarter of four." It was five-thirty now. He say to the nurse, "And you say she just got here?" And she say, "*Uh—uh—uh!*" "Almost two hours?" he said. "And you didn't call me?" "I didn't think it was time." Oh, I said, Lord have mercy. Now I say if I had to go back under *that* nurse, I don't think I would go to the hospital.

Why do you not want to have it at home? Did you have any trouble the first birth?

Oh! That's another reason why. He say I have a tendency to have high blood pressure when I get pregnant.

How old were you when you had your first child?

I think I was twenty-two.

Do you remember your most vivid memory about that one?

Well, that one I couldn't tell; I cut so much "G" with that one. [Laughter.] Oh, boy! I just went *on* and *on*. I told my mother, "I'm gonna die." I say, "Well, never no more! I don't want to *see* another one." My mother told me, "Oh, you just saying that." I say, "*No,* I don't wanna see another one."

The midwife didn't help you, tell you not to worry?

She helped me, she helped me. She said, "If you will just bear with the pains, this child is just about here. The main thing is," she say, "you don't have nothin' to worry about." But I think they pitied me a lot. [Laughter.] When he came, I said, "Lord!" and then I start laughing. I say, "Willie." She say, "Now that was a trip for you. If you hadn't been so spoiled, you woulda had an easy time." She said, "But ja' mama just done spoiled ya." [Laughter.]

Your mother was there babying you?

Yeah. Oh, and I was laying on her lap and was saying I didn't wanta stay in bed; I wanted to get up in her lap. If I hadda really knowed what to do, I . . .

What about the second time?

The second time I kinda had a hard time 'cause I hurt myself with that child, and he was stillborn. [Long silence.]

What about the third?

Well, my third one. *Oh, boy!* That was hot peas! [She shudders.] I was in labor when my water broke. I think it was a day or two before the child came. And my cousin happened to been to the house, and I was up to my sister-in-law's. I saw that child, and he turned around, and it was good, but I didn't know what it was doin'. And it stretched and, "Ugh!" punched so hard I jumped. And my sister-in-law said, "Oooh, look at that baby!" She say, "You gonna have that baby. You ain't goin' to the house. That child done dropped; he almost here." My husband came up there, and so I walked on back with him. I got there to the house and sat on the bed. I had got up that day, washed; I mopped my house right; I ironed my clothes; I even took and changed the linens off the bed that I'd slept on and washed 'em all up. And oh, I had cleaned my pot, oh, everything! I had all my dish towels all scalded and hanging up. There was two men came to the house, and we was sitting in the house talking. And I was sitting up on the bed. "Look!" I say, "Oh, my goodness. You better do something!" I told Sam.

That's your husband?

Yeah. And I stood up in the water. I said, "Oooh, what in the world in here?" I just start to crying. I thought I done kill the baby. But she said, "How you know?" I said, "I *know* it." She said, "What is *this?* Well, I ain't never. . . ." So, I went out in the yard, and we had a outta-doors toilet. I said, "Oooh, I got to go out here in this toilet." And she say, "*You* better not to go out there!" Well, I say, "I got to wet." She say, "Well, you better not to go out there." But I went. And I looked at him right, and I said, "Lord, have mercy, how stupid I was." And I just looked at him and shook my head. Every time he come home, I have to look and think about it, what a narrow escape he was. [Laughter.] Oh, I done some miserable things. Somebody asked me, "Had you told him

about it?" I said, "No, that's *one* of the things I ain't a gonna tell him."
I won't let him know I was that stupid.

At your births there were never any men in the room?

Hmmm, well, wait a minute. No, I think Sam come in there with
that *first* child. But I was cuttin' all kinda 'Gs" over it. "I'm not letting
Sam in there," I said. I told 'em I didn't want him in there. [The mid-
wife] say, "Somebody said you better not come in here, Sam." She say,
"Why?" I say, "*I don't want him in here!*" I say, "This will be the *last*
child!" And so, she say, "Come on, push 'em." I say, "I'm comin' because this'll be your last one!" She say, "What you gettin' mad with
him about?" I say, "I *mean* it!" I don't see how they got this thing. It
looked like to me I had a hard pain once or twice, and I just couldn't
make it. She say, "Well, if you let your husband come . . ." I say, "Well,
not yet, I'll try it again." I tried and tried, and with that last try, I said,
"Okay," I say, "let him come in." I say, "Y'all know that's the biggest
mess I ever been in. Well," I say, "I'm kinda embarrassed." [Laughter.] I
said, "Don't come in here *lookin'* at me!"

Did they think that he would calm you down and help you?

I don't even know, 'cause I think maybe that they announced that he
was coming in [was] what hit 'em; he was there, and Gerald say,
"*Waaaaa!*" Sam say, "Good Lord!" [Laughter.] She say, "Oooh, you
gotta [boy]. This is a little Samuel, Junior."

Right when he came in, the baby was born?

Reckon it was by the time he got in there. He say, "Well, I sure got
my wishes; I wanted a boy." She say, "Well, you got your little Samuel,

Junior." And I say, "Lord, I wanted a girl *so* bad." But Sam wanted the boy, so I had to settle for the boy.

Did you have any daughters?

[Shakes her head no.]

Why did you want a daughter?

I think a girl in some ways is more sensitive to her mother. For instance, if I get sick, my daughter could be there to kinda wait on me.

You don't think a son would do that?

Well, I won't say they can't do just like a daughter, but I would rather a daughter. I used to work with this white lady, and she had children, two sons and a daughter. They was grown, two of 'em married out, and the younger one was her son, her youngest son. And she fell and broke her hip. He took care of her just like if she was a little baby. He'd give her her bath. She says, "Oh, Jenny, I hate so bad for him to have to look all over me." I say, "Well, just don't say nothin' about it. Just thank the good Lord that he is nice enough to do it." I say, "And I don't think he mind it." She say, "I don't either, but, I just hate for him to look over me like *this*." I say, "Well, you can't help it." And I would offer to give her her medicine and all. I mean, oh Lord, sometimes I almost slipped—now, I don't know whether I would want my son to do *this* or not.

How many women were there with you at the first birth?

My mother . . .

Was your grandmother there?

No, my grandmother—I think she had just passed on or she got sick. And my cousin. Just three people.

And was your midwife there that night?

Yeah, just three *with* the midwife.

When you go through something like that with those women, do you feel closer to them?

Well, you sure do. I guess that's what's got me mixed up like that. 'Cause this midwife, I always thought there wouldn't be another one like her. And I never did . . .

What was she like?

She was nice.

Was she very spiritual?

Yeah, oh yes, my goodness. She even had her little Bible to read the Scriptures. Once she read the Twenty-third Psalm. And she read another one—I think it was in the Psalms, too. I think it was the Thirty-fifth—I'm not sure. Or the Twenty-seventh.

Things that would give you comfort? How long would she sit up with you like that?

Right there till the end. Sometimes, you know, she'd stretch out. There was two little twin beds, and now and then she would lay down on the bed. I kinda liked that. I know they give you better attention in the home . . . when you're all alone.

So she delivered all your babies except for the last one?

And that woman—that was my mother's midwife. She waited on my mother for all of us.

How old was she when she died?

Oh, it was ninety-something.

Was she delivering right up until she died?

I don't think so. She was eighty probably before she stopped. Oh, and she was so patient! She was a *nice* person.

Did you ever think about the biblical story of Eve and what it had to do with your births?

Well, you mean wedlock?

Whatever you want to say.

I ain't too sure about that. They say the Lord puts you here *for* that, but maybe there's a time for it. Now, I think they should be married. That's the way I feel about it. *I* was married, I know. I don't think I'd a been livin' now if I'd a had one 'fore I was married. My mother used to tell us all the time, "Don't bring no child that ain't born in wedlock." Oh, but I'm not too in favor of it. I think they *should* get married.

Would your midwife deliver girls whether they were married or not?

Now, I don't know about that. I guess she did. I can't say she did and I can't say she didn't. Because all she delivered, I know *they* was married. But that don't say she didn't deliver more.

Do you remember anything after your first child that changed your way of looking at yourself, something that surprised you about yourself?

I don't think so.

Did you know you had that much strength—physical strength?

Oooh, I sure didn't. I really didn't. And I used to think about that sometime, and I'll draw up after the child was born. After the first child came, I was, for a long time, 'cause he was a big baby. I just think about it [she shudders], just like that. Think about things—oooh! Oooh!

The second one was a stillborn? You had real hard experiences the first two times.

That child. You know, I took a douche, but I didn't know you can't take no douche. Nobody never told me, and I don't know how my first child here. I guess the Lord take care all fools. 'Cause I took the douche from the time I learned how to take the douche till it almost got here.

What was it?

Let me see, I think it was a tablespoon of vinegar in warm water. I'm not sure. Was it vinegar? I'm not sure what I took—if it were vinegar. Sometimes I had the water kinda warm. That particular time, they say the water was *too* warm, and I drowned the child, and I scalded it. Lord!

So you think that's why the second child was stillborn?

'Cause one side of its face was blue-like. Oh, Lord have mercy, Jesus. I had to go to the doctor, and the doctor had to cut. She say I might have to have treatment. [Long pause. She is looking down.]

Let me ask you about breast-feeding. How do you feel when you see a young woman breast-feeding nowadays?

I think it's great 'cause I breast-fed my children.

Some people feel offended by it when it's done in public.

Oh, well, now, I always tried to go in a kinda place; if not, if I can't get a kind of private place, I always carried me a little hand towel. I didn't just stick my breast out there in public.

Why do you think women stopped breast-feeding for a while?

Well, I think sometimes some people just don't want their children nursing the breast 'cause they pull the breasts down and make 'em look bad.

What do you see as a woman's greatest problem in this world?

Oh, I don't know about that. I guess just trying to make it through this here world. [Laughter.] Oh, goodness, I don't know—so *many* problems! Maybe trying to make ends meet, for one. Oh, gosh, paying all these expensive bills with no money hardly.

*   *   *   *   *

You had all sons?

Sons! My three sons. [Laughter.]

How many grandchildren?

Five.

Any girls there?

Yes, two girls.

How old is your oldest girl?

The oldest girl is twenty-three.

Do you have a close relationship with her?

Well, yes and no. These young folks, they so *wild!* She's alright, but she's kinda high-strung. She want to have her way. Some folks raise their children different. And well, I guess my children say I'm old-fashioned. I just don't like all this here stuff that you young folks doin'. Me and her haves it out sometimes. [Laughter.]

The only question I have left is whether you found anything spiritual about childbirthing.

Any special about who?

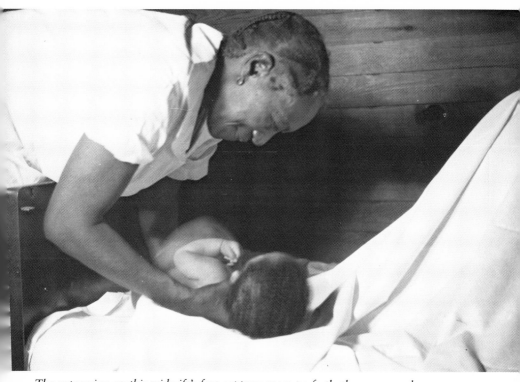

The expression on this midwife's face captures more perfectly than any words the spirit and love of the women who served as midwives.

Midwives often attended childbirth in the worst of conditions but impressively with no higher infant and maternal mortality rates than physicians. County health nurses and midwives would venture into deep-woods rural areas to reach women in need of assistance. The photographs here were taken in the early 1930s.

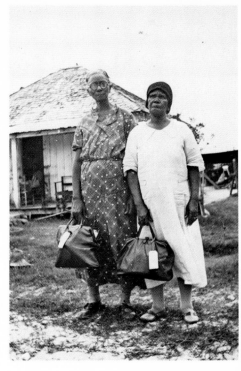

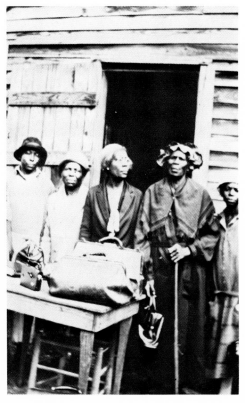

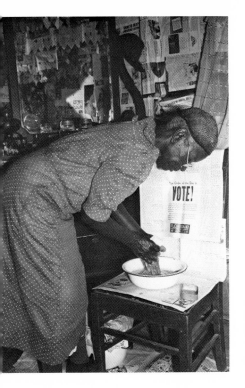

County health training encouraged the use of a sterile and well-equipped midwife's bag. The midwife was adept at creating her own sterile environment when one could not be provided, as these photographs of a midwife in 1944 show. As most of the midwife's "clients" lived in poverty, her desire to practice was necessarily removed from any material motive and was rooted in a spiritual "calling" and love for her work.

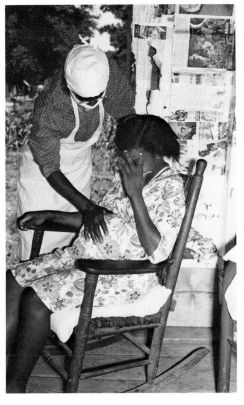

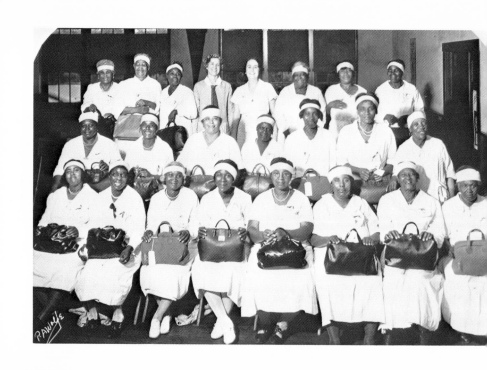

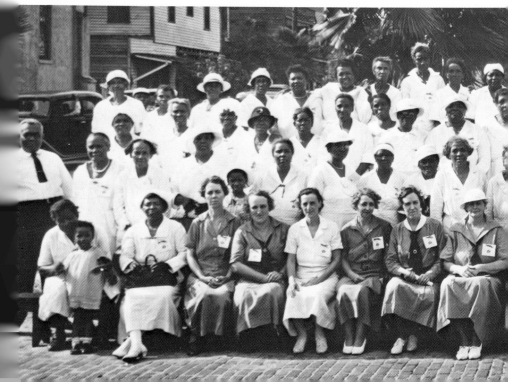

Midwife institutes were held regionally around Florida, attracting midwives from the surrounding area for a week of instruction on aseptic birth procedures. A "certificate of fitness" was awarded to those who completed the course and could display a clean and properly equipped midwife's bag. The certificate carried with it no legal significance and attendance at the institutes was not required, but the midwives' response to these seminar-workshops was strong and positive. The groups shown here are from institutes in St. Augustine (left) and Tampa (below) in 1934 and 1935, respectively.

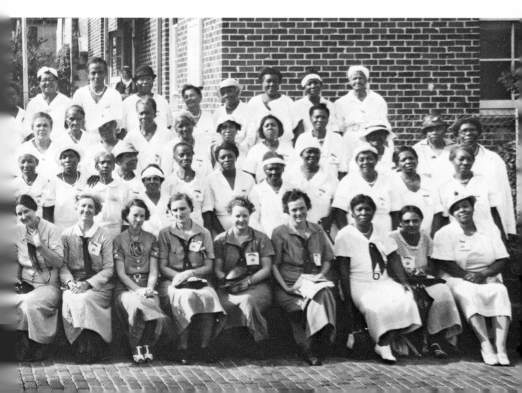

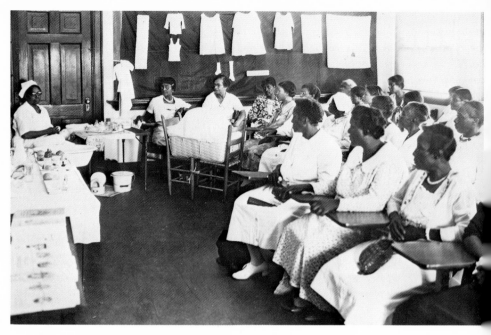

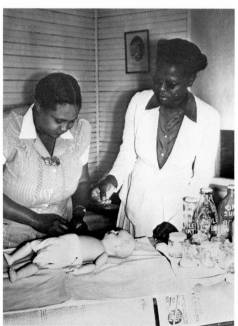

Classes such as this one in child nutrition (above)—given at the midwife institute at Florida A&M University, Tallahassee, in 1935—were offered by the state for thirteen years. In 1946 the midwife institutes were permanently discontinued, and jurisdiction for the supervision of midwives shifted from the state to the county level (left). "Young colored nurses of pleasing personality," usually coming from the northern United States, were sought to supervise local midwives.

ese young nurses administered state policies
the county level; they held classes on
eptic birth procedures, taught midwives
w to fill out birth certificates, and
nducted periodic inspections of the
dwives' bags.

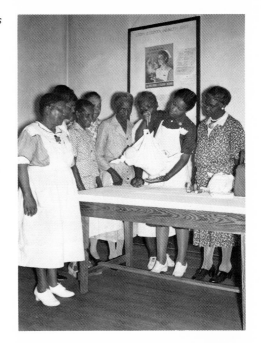

Miss Chase" (below) was the invention of
le Graves, the Florida state supervisory
rse of midwives until the late 1940s. The
e-size birthing mannequin was used in
nulated birth instruction. She came
mplete with trapdoor abdomen, baby,
nbilical cord, and placenta and was
signed to be marketed as either a black or
hite model.

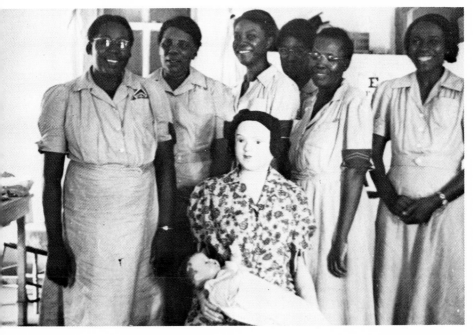

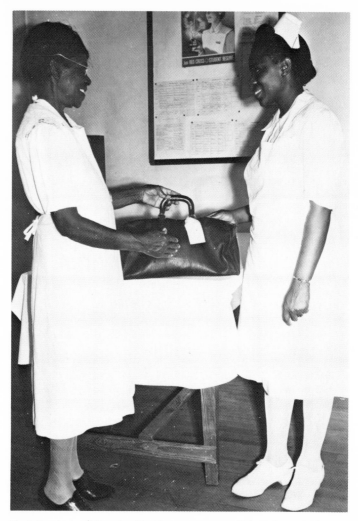

Training in traditional midwifery was accomplished through the apprenticeship model, usually passed on within the same family. In their efforts to persuade traditional midwives to give up their practice, the State Board of Health employed this model, substituting young black, hospital-trained nurses in the apprentice/trainee role. The older midwife was expected to surrender her midwife's bag to her "young protégée—thereby removing the temptation to take an occasional case."

*Spiritual—anything spiritual about birthing children. It's real phys-
ical, but do you remember having any thoughts or feelings about that
or thinking about your grandmother and things she'd been through or
all the women of the world . . .*

Oh, yes! Yeah, I used to do it. I think about that a lot now. But all
these memories just comes back to me. Really, some of these things I
just don't think I'll forget. And then sometimes I can think of things
that happened a long time ago better than I can things that happened
just recently. 'Cause somebody could tell me something here today, and
I'd soon forget it. Oh, sometimes I get so upset with myself, I don't
know what to do.

Is your husband still alive?

He's dead.

Have you ever remarried?

No. Don't *plan* to. [Laughter.]

Why not?

I just don't. Then again, I have seen these stepfathers and step-
mothers, how they treat the children. And I don't want to go to jail.
And I don't want to be a murderer. Course, I wouldn't have to be one
now 'cause the children could take care of themselves. But I don't want
no man over my children. Mm-hmm, I used to live right next to a
couple, and that man—that was enough for me. I said, never. I told my
husband when he came home that day, "If anything would happen to
you, I *never* put a man over my children." I said, "If anything to hap-

pen to me first, *please* don't put no woman over my children." He laughed. He said, "Well, by the time I be dead, you be . . ." I said, "No, siree."

Were any of your children still at home when he died?

Yeah, they was home.

Was that hard being alone then?

Yes, it was hard, but, oh, I took it on . . .

How many years had you been married?

My youngest wasn't born yet. I didn't even know I was pregnant, but I was *thinking* I was.

Was it hard to carry the baby without him?

It was. Yes, 'cause I worried a lot, and I grieved a lot. I cried a lot.

Did you think about him when you were having it?

I sure did. And when I hear that he was a boy, I said, "Oh, Lord."

You got through a lot, didn't you?

Sure do. The good Lord will take care of us.

Interview with Johnnie Seeley and Company,
April 1982

This is a group interview including all the participants
at the birth of Nellie Jean, the daughter of a white
middle-class couple who took their birth across county
lines in order to employ the only legal midwife in the
area. That midwife was Johnnie Seeley, a black woman
who has delivered a couple thousand babies and, due
to a bad hip, now delivers exclusively in her rural
north-Florida home. The parents are Victoria, who
hails from Great Britain, and her husband Robert. A
friend and nursing student, Marlena, was also present
to assist.

*Why don't we start by having each of you tell us your most memora-
ble moment of the day Nellie Jean was born.*

Johnnie: She don't know. The most exciting moment [was] when I
told her I saw the head. That was the most exciting. [Laughter.] When I
saw it: "I see the head!"

Victoria: Yeah. I think that was it: when it was actually pushed out
and I could see it there before Nellie actually came out of my body.
What about for you, Robert?

Robert: Oh, I'd have to concur. That's the peak, when it starts to
come out. Because you've been working so hard and waiting for it and
hoping it would come out, come out, come out, come out . . .

How about you, Johnnie? You've gone through so many.

Johnnie: I'm so used to it. They all come out the same.

Let's start talking about the birth and everyone just jump in when you want to continue the story. [Marlena has just entered the room. You missed the question about what part of the birth was the most exciting. What was it for you?

Marlena: For me? The most exciting? Oh, goodness, when the head came out. [Everyone laughs.]

Everyone has said that.

Marlena: Oh, it's just incredible. Oh, it was.

Johnnie: She said, "Oh! I've never been this close to one before."

Marlena: Well, always at the hospital you have to stand back fifteen feet. I would be with women in the labor room and then go over to the delivery room with them, but the doctor comes and takes over and you have to kind of stand back. I would blueprint the baby and help out the mother and do prep work and everything. But when the doctor's delivering, you have to stand back. It's six to ten feet back.

You mean they actually tell you how far to stand back?

Marlena: Oh, no, I'm just saying approximately. You just make sure you're well enough out of the way 'cause people are scurrying around. You have to be more than just four feet in back of him 'cause people got to get around the doctor; so you got to be a little further back. I was up on the bed against the wall on one side and he [Robert] was sittin' on half of the bed on the other side.

What exactly was everyone doing while you were in labor; what were your roles; how were you helping?

Johnnie: Well, she was gettin' the paper ready, gettin' the white sheet tear paper off to have it ready for me when I need it. Keep her face wet down. There was little things that she could do to try to keep comfortable.

Marlena: For a while, before she went through transition where the head was really ready to come out, she was down on the floor, and Robert was rubbing her back mainly. I was timing contractions, and Johnnie was encouraging her and checking on her, head to toe. And the contractions—when we got here, they were two or three minutes apart, but then they went up, back up to five and six minutes apart for a couple of hours; and then they started coming down back to two and three minutes apart. And that was right around the transition time. You can usually tell that because mainly what women will say is, "I feel like I have to have a bowel movement." Because there is so much pressure, that's what they think they want to do. They need to have that urge to really push. By the next contraction, we had her up on the bed. Mainly, that's what we were doing. And in between I was crocheting a little thing for her—mainly talking with Victoria.

So then the whole birth from the time you got here took about four hours?

Marlena: Four.

No complications?

Johnnie: No complications whatever.

When it slowed down when she first got here, is that just adjusting to a new place?

Johnnie: No, it just happens that way.

Marlena: Usually I've found, with you or for other people, that it never really goes back up past five or six minutes unless something *is* wrong. But with her, it just went up to six minutes. Once it came down, it just came back right down.

Can you describe how you first felt, Victoria, when you first saw Nellie Jean?

Victoria: Well, I remember being surprised that she was a girl because everybody had said I was gonna have a little boy. But my first things I thought that I would feel—I thought that I'd feel very motherly, you know, seeing my baby, but I didn't feel that way at all. It was just like, "Who is this little person that I just—that just popped out?" It was a wonderful feeling, though, to see her there, to see her look around. But I didn't feel as motherly straightaway as I thought I would. It was like a little stranger.

When did that come, feeling motherly?

Victoria: Probably a couple of days later when I'd relaxed and got used to her.

Do you remember any recurring thoughts you had during the labor itself?

Victoria: I remember it not being as hard as I thought it was going to be. I was waiting for it to get harder than it was. I thought that I was gonna go through more pain than I did. I remember thinking that if this is how it's gonna be, it's okay, but if it's gonna get *more* painful, it's *not* gonna be okay. But it didn't.

Marlena: It was just right.

Victoria: Yeah.

Here's a question for Robert: Is there anything you learned about yourself or Victoria during that time that you were surprised to find out?

Robert: That I was *surprised* to find out?

Or that you learned, that you didn't know before?

Robert: Patience. It's just a matter of developing patience, different rhythms, different expectations. It changes your style of living, and every alteration you make in that style takes a little adjustment.

Did either of you feel surprised at the amount of strength you displayed in labor?

Robert: No.

Victoria: No. Because, like I said, I thought I was gonna have to use *more* strength than I ever had before.

You had some on reserve.

Victoria: Yeah.

Upon the birth of her first son, Queen Victoria's eldest daughter was reported to have said, "It is hard indeed to be separated from one's own mother when one has only just learnt what one owes her." What are your reactions to that?

Victoria: In fact, yeah. I didn't have my mother there because my mother's in England. Having such a new little baby, I didn't really know everything that I'm supposed to do with it. I didn't know how to do this or that, and a mother would have been very helpful then to help out.

How about this one from Kathleen Cleaver, who was married to Eldridge Cleaver: "I've become a mother. That's why women grow up and men don't."

Robert: Well, I can see there's a point to that question. Having a child can certainly radically change your life for a woman much more so than for a man because she has to [baby cries block out voice]. What I was saying was that I think it binds you together in a certain way depending on the attitude you take. I feel a great deal of commitment to Nellie, and I don't think that a woman has any right to say that it's her child and that she is the one who is totally responsible for it, by any means.

Do you want to comment on that quote?

Marlena: I don't know, 'cause I think there's a change in the male and female roles, that the men *are* more involved now than when that quote was written, but I'm not sure. I don't know enough about the history of that woman. That was still a time when men didn't do what Robert did, either. They weren't helping their wives have the babies so much as they do now.

Johnnie, what was your mother like?

Johnnie: My mother was like a pretty good housewife, she was a good cook, she didn't—well, she worked out, but mostly she stayed at home, kept the house, she sewed, did some sewing and made quilts and things like that. She was kind of a quiet person to me; you know I'm going to say she was good 'cause she was my mother. Of course, she wasn't a midwife, but her mother, my grandmother, was. But that still didn't entice me.

How'd you become a midwife?

Johnnie: Well, a lady lived down the street there. She was a midwife, and she'd gotten old. She said, "I'm gettin' old; somebody got to take it." I'd been with her several times, and she just kept on asking me about joinin' the board, but I didn't *want* to be a midwife. So I kept pushin' her off until at last, one day, my grandson was born here. My daughter had her baby okay; she sits back and lets me deliver the baby. I did the cord and everything and dressed the baby. The old midwife looked at me and laughed. She said, "Why don't you come on and go to the meetin' Friday?" I said, "I will." I'd be gettin' her off my back, you know. She kept so closely; I said, "Well, I'm goin'." So really that Friday I went, and after I joined the board, then everywhere she went, every time she got a call, she would call me 'cause I was drivin' a car. And she would go on and call me and tell me to come where she was. And I did that. In a year's time, I had got my license. At that time, you could go under the supervision of another midwife until you get, I think it was, fifteen deliveries; or you could be supervised by a doctor. At that time, the doctors [would come out], but you can't get no doctor out now. I went under the supervision of a midwife. And in a year's time, I got my license. First, the nurse come up from Jacksonville and give you these tests and find out what you know, and see if you [inaudible due to baby cries] put in for your license 'cause they come from Jacksonville.

How old were you when you started?

Johnnie: I was, hmm, thirty-seven when I started.

Did they make a special rule for G—— County? Because that new law is up before the Florida house again. And it doesn't say anything about your doing it under a midwife, but that you have to have a physician.

Johnnie: See, what they're sayin', there's a nurse-midwife which works in the hospital—no, maybe they work in the [rural areas?] too. I don't know. At one time, they was tryin' to get one here to work in the hospital, but that still wouldn't interfere with the lay midwives working out in the rural. So I don't know what's gonna happen. We was talkin' about that down at the health department this morning. Miss M—— said they're gonna have this hearing, and she wanted to recommend two of us to go.

Really? It passed the Florida senate yesterday.

Johnnie: I wouldn't mind goin', whenever they had the meetings. But you see, all she could do was send in a recommendation. It's up to the governor to appoint who was to go. So I don't know what they're gonna do about it. Every once in a while they put something in the paper about it. But this is my idea, now: I'm thinkin' midwives gonna be around for a long time. I say from now on around in G—— County 'cause they say G—— County is one of the richest counties in the world. But there's a lot of people here not able to go to the hospital 'cause ain't nobody hardly can afford to go to the hospital now, the way they are. But now here's another thing. There's a lot of *unwed* mothers, and some got husbands. They on welfare, and they go to hospital and have their baby, see, and the welfare pays for them. Now Reagan's gonna cut so much offa the budget; why don't he cut those seven to eight hundred dollars—maybe a thousand dollars—that they payin' for a woman to go to the hospital and have a baby. See, now lookin' at that, yet they want to come around here maybe cut somebody's Social Security, cut off the medicare. But there's where he need to cut it.

And then have them come to midwives?

Johnnie: Yeah. He could do that. But they don't see it. One of the welfare workers called me to get some information, and I asked him. He said, "You know what? That never has been brought up." So I think it would be worthwhile to mention. Maybe they *would* pay. 'Cause they pay the doctor in the hospital, but they won't pay a midwife. It may be because it never has been brought up.

Or maybe because the doctors don't want it.

Johnnie: They *don't* want it 'cause, see, they don't deliver those babies, but they get paid. And he wants his money before that baby's born. You pay him, and they want you to pay the hospital. So they say no problem; they admit you right on in the hospital.

Legislators were asking for midwives to go to college and get a nursing degree rather than to apprentice like you did. We were asking, "Why go to nursing school when only a small part of that four years is devoted to obstetrics?"

Marlena: Only because it gives you a medical background.

They seemed to have little knowledge of or respect for lay midwifery.

Marlena: Well, because they have what I call a professional attitude, and it's a fixed entity of the fact that if it's in laymen's terms, then it's not a profession. If it's a profession, then you're dealing with someone's life. Somehow it's not as safe. I could be wrong, but where ninety percent of pregnancies are trouble free, it's like three or four percent of women who know beforehand they're gonna have problems. The reason they say "precarious" is because a woman who is pregnant *can* develop problems during the pregnancy even though it doesn't *normally* happen. It can happen, and it can be an emergency situation. The basis of their fear to have people go to the hospital is that medicine treats anything like a disease, and it can treat pregnancy like a disease. What is the risk? When a woman who is in the middle of her labor goes into an emergency or gets problems, it's usually more of an emergency situation and requires immediate care. And their contention is that possibly the medical background would afford this person even to know how to do emergency medical techniques. I don't say this is right, because this woman *obviously* knows what she is doing.

Johnnie: The nurse—she still can't deliver babies without her midwife license.

Marlena: Unless it's an emergency.

Johnnie: That's right.

EMTs and paramedics who drive ambulances are not required to have a college degree, and they do far more than a midwife. They're also constantly dealing with emergency situations of life and death. And yet the legislators don't see that if you let EMTs practice without a four-year degree, why not a midwife who does this one special thing?

Marlena: But they're not trying to take over the doctor's job. [Laughter.] People just get it in their minds that if you don't learn it via a school, you haven't learned it somehow. That's *their* ignorance. I call it an overeducated ignorance. I'm sure there are some midwives that may need a refresher course, but there are a lot of doctors and nurses that need that, too. I just think that when you learn something like what Johnnie's learned and you do it pretty much on an everyday basis . . .

Passing down of knowledge from mother to daughter is also getting lost here. We don't think that way anymore. We send ourselves to schools, and this person we've never met before teaches these things.

Marlena: The United States is rated as one of the top fifteen countries with the worst medical services. It's rated like fifteen for sure. Considering how many countries there are in the world and how many are underdeveloped, to have such—well, that's just medicine in general. It boils down to poor people can't afford health care, first of all, just in overall generalized medicine. And as far as obstetrics goes, people who become pregnant, especially if they're unwed mothers, I think that they don't get the care that they need. Not necessarily during labor and delivery; it's—

Johnnie: Before labor—prenatal.

Marlena: Right. The prenatal care. They end up with complications because they didn't get proper prenatal care, and a lot of it is because they couldn't afford it. Those funds are not available. So it's not the midwife's fault a lot of the time. You could say that sometimes that blame gets put there when it shouldn't be. I think a lot of that has to do with that they may have lacked prenatal care beforehand, especially young mothers who are still growing themselves. They encounter physical problems because of their age.

Let me ask you, Johnnie, do you think there's a difference in the young mothers now who are choosing to stay at home and birth and the mothers who stayed at home and birthed during your time?

Johnnie: No. There's no difference. There's no difference about 'em staying home. Now, I'll tell you why. The most of those that go to the hospital, they're goin' on the welfare. You know, these young mothers. That's why they go to the hospitals. If it weren't for the welfare paying the bill, *they* would be stayin' home. So there's no difference.

I'm wondering about the cultural difference between blacks and whites. My mother's generation didn't even consider staying home. It was the thing to do to go to the hospital. There's a difference between the way our grandmothers stayed at home when everyone did it and the way young women stay home in T——, where it would be illegal to do it.

Johnnie: It may have been for the simple reason that they didn't have any midwives is why *they* went, see. Just like in T——, a lot of those people would stay home, but they just don't have any midwives. That's why they go to the hospital. They don't go because they *prefer* to go. A lot of them would rather stay home, but they just have to go.

How'd it get to this point? Why did we all start going to the hospital?

Johnnie: I don't know *why* they all went unless they was in a county that didn't use midwives. That could have been the problem. They could have been in Florida and still been livin' in a county that didn't use midwives.

Where did the midwives go?

Johnnie: I don't know where they went. Well, I know where *ours* went. Some died, some retired, so that leaves us with four. When I started bein' a midwife in 1960, we had fourteen in G—— County. Some—well, most of 'em—died, and there's three or four of 'em retired. You take right there in B——, they *use* midwives, but they don't have any. I guess the midwives just vanished somewhere.

They're not passing it down anymore.

Johnnie: They must not be, 'cause they really don't have any. I've had several people come from down there. I told them to stop; I'm not ramblin' way down in B—— to deliver no babies. I'll go to G——, and I don't care about goin' there, I used to go to C—— and everywhere, but I told 'em I'm not doing that anymore. I ain't goin' to C——; I ain't goin' to H——. And *not* to B——. If you all want to come to my house, that's well and good, but I'm not comin' down there. It's too far.

How did you feel about your body, Victoria, as it grew bigger and changed?

Victoria: I really enjoyed being pregnant. I really enjoyed the experience. It felt wonderful to me to have that life inside of you. And just how it changed all the time and by the end how big it was. How your body, how your skin stretches, how it contains that baby in there. Feeling it moving, the baby moving. I really enjoyed that. I felt really good; I felt very healthy. It was a good time for me.

Did you feel any different psychologically?

Victoria: I'm sure. I'm sure there must have been. That probably went along with the physical thing of, as I got bigger, not being able to do certain things. I'd have to change my attitude. I was frustrated now and again at *not* being able to do certain things.

I saw you riding your bike right to the end.

Victoria: Yeah. I was riding my bike to about seven—

Marlena: Just the end of your sixth month.

Do you think that helped her—the bicycle riding?

Johnnie: Mm-hmm.

Victoria: I got more exercise then than I do now. [Laughter.]

Did you feel any kind of letdown feeling after birth?

Victoria: No. I had heard that some women do feel that, but I didn't feel that way at all. I mean, I felt very tired some days, but I didn't feel letdown or depressed.

Johnnie, could you relate one of the most unusual births you've ever attended? How many babies have you delivered?

Johnnie: Well, it's more than two thousand. I once had it counted about two years ago. Some of the most exciting deliveries I've ever had was twins when the mother don't really know they're gonna have twins. I had one, a niece, she was very small. Had twins—two boys. Of course, she didn't know she was gonna have any twins. And when the first one came, I laid the baby over there. The mother's still layin' there. She said, "Well, somethin's scratchin' me!" [Laughter.] I said, "Nothin's scratchin' you." "Yes, it is! Well, what is it?" So I looked at her, and said, "You're gonna have another 'un." "Oh!" She just went to cryin', "What am I gonna do with two babies?" [Laughter.] I said, "Now wait a minute. You ain't had him yet." The first one came, you know, head first. The last one came, he stuck one hand out like that [sticks fist out], and then stick his head down and his feet came out. But it just come on out; we didn't have no problems. But she just went to cryin' when I told her there was another baby there. "I don't want no two babies!" [Laughter.] They got big-size little boys now, and they's just runnin' all over everywhere.

What was Johnnie's bedside manner like?

Marlena: Wonderful.

Victoria: Wonderful. [Laughter.]

Can you be more specific?

Robert: No nonsense. Stayed cool.

Marlena: Cool, calm, and very supportive. Very encouraging.

Victoria: I remember one time when I was on the bed, I just started pushin', and Johnnie says to me, "Shut your mouth!" [Laughter.] Then I realized that she meant put my energy down there instead of out here.

Johnnie: For her to close her mouth so he could come down through.

Marlena: She was confident and sure.

You never felt like anything was going to go wrong?

Victoria: Oh, no, no. Not under Johnnie's care. Not at all.

How about eye contact? How much talk and how much nonverbal communication goes on?

Victoria: I remember we seemed to have talked a lot. You were having some good conversations.

Marlena: When you were on the floor, we had more nonchalant conversations.

Did you feel like talking?

Victoria: Oh, yeah, just before I got on the bed, yeah. In fact, all the way through I felt like . . .

Robert: Well, in the latter stages you weren't doin' much talking, 'cause you were workin' too hard.

Marlena: And then once you're on the bed, we'd be down at the end saying, "Okay, lay straight, push down, breathe this way, you know, keep your—

Victoria: And I'd be askin' questions like, "Can you see it yet?" [Laughter.]

Since you didn't know Victoria that well before the birth, and you've said your relationship with her has taken on a different aspect, can you explain what the differences are?

Marlena: It was, first of all, the fact that we were going to be doin' a home delivery as opposed to a hospital delivery. All of us personally felt that we should get to know each other as well as we can, because when you're actually goin' through the birth, you have to feel confident and comfortable and secure with the people that you're with. I wasn't really required to spend as much time as I did, but the first night actually that you and I—we, all of us—got together and had dinner before we actually made a final decision, I knew within like five minutes of talkin' with Robert that I just wanted to be able to be there and to get to know them, and I know they wanted to get to know me. It was just this natural clicking in. And we just hit it off so beautifully that we found that we could all communicate well together, so that when the time actually did come, we would know what to do with each other. I found that especially as the time got closer, I just started really feeling an attachment towards not only the baby but to Victoria and Robert. Everybody was close—it was like brothers and sisters. That's kinda how I—yeah, that's how I feel. The closer she got to her [due date], the more excited I even got about it. It was just more like a family thing. We all went through it together, and we all kinda shared the load. It was easy to do because we all knew that we could rely upon each other in that way. And it's been that way ever since. It's my goddaughter in there. [Laughter.] It's been the formation of some of the best relationships I've ever had in my life. You know, it's as close as I am with my own family, which I'm real close to.

Do you remember how you were feeling toward Victoria during the labor itself?

Marlena: Yeah, I felt really connected with you; I felt a good connection between all of us and just a lot of love, and I wanted her to be as comfortable as possible and to help her through it in any way that I could. A lot of times I found that was either by assisting Johnnie or, when she would be going through a pushing contraction, to talk her through it. I don't know if it helped any or if she even heard . . .

Victoria: I was holding your arm . . .

Marlena: That's right, we were holding hands. I was sitting on the end of the bed. We held hands through the last twenty minutes or so. She didn't want to let go of my hand. She felt that support was needed, and so I gave it, and Robert—she was holding Robert on the other end, and I was up there holding. We were both pulling on the side. [Laughter.] I was holding back one of her legs and holding her hand; we were just like we had eight arms all of a sudden, and you do seem to have arms to do everything you need to do.

Why don't we just go around and let everyone say one final remark on birthing in general or this birth in particular.

Victoria: Did you want to know my reasons why I chose a midwife?

I want to hear anything you want to tell me.

Victoria: I'd decided that I wanted a midwife basically because I'm scared of the hospital. I felt that hospitals are for sick people, and that's where you go. Or if I was gonna have any complications, I would have gone to a hospital; but if everything was gonna be okay, I felt it would be better for me to have a midwife because I'd be more relaxed. Therefore, the baby would come out better than if I was in the hospital in such unnatural surroundings where I *knew* I'd just be tense, really tense.

Did it work?

Victoria: Yeah, it worked wonderfully.

Robert: Well, I suppose I was really impressed by the pure natural logic about it, the body having a nine-month gestation period. It really gave us *all* time to be prepared for the event. I mean, when you first think about it at month two or three or one and a half, whenever you plan to have the baby, you start considering alternatives. The idea of having the baby at home or with a midwife or wherever is a little bit horrifying at first, 'cause you don't know that much about it. But once you have lots and lots of time to investigate and plan for it and get used to the idea and think about it and talk about it, when it happens, you're prepared for it. You know, people like fathers who keep thinkin' about it are scared to death at the thought of being able to be there and participate. You've got all that time to prepare for it. You see, it's not something you'd *want* to have happen like that [snaps fingers], because you *wouldn't* be prepared for it. It's all very, very natural.

Marlena: I think that the whole process of delivering babies—as far as between doing it at home or doing it in a clinical setting, not even a hospital per se, but maybe a midwifery clinic—I agree with what Victoria has said. I think that hospitals are just as necessary as the midwives are—mainly by the fact that the people who, first of all, have the physical problems that show up while they're going through their prenatal period, those people *need* a hospital. They need the emergency attention. Those people *are* higher risk; they need that type of clinical setting. The people who psychologically feel better or safer in a hospital *need* the clinical setting. The people who are in excellent health and really don't show the fact that they're going to have a problem to have it at home—if they psychologically feel that's what they want, then they should be in their home or in a midwife's home. Whatever surroundings put the mother in the least type of danger—and that includes a psychological outlook—it's very important. I think stress wears the mother out; it causes more pain. If they feel insecure, they're not going to relax; it's gonna make it a longer, harder delivery. So if she is going to feel unsafe out of the hospital, she should be in a hospital. I think that the only thing I would say about midwives and doing it at home is that where there is the possibility of an emergency arising within a pregnancy situation, being in a house where a hospital is close by would be the ideal thing.

Of course, you need doctors that are receptive.

Marlena: That's my personal ideal, but it depends on wherever it's psychologically and helpfully most secure for that person in particular; that's where they should be. But I do tend to think that more women would probably have babies at home if it was more accepted that they could go to the hospital in case there was an emergency.

Victoria: I had some people be horrified when I said I had a home delivery; some mothers were really horrified. They thought that was terrible. I know one person thinking that it was terribly selfish of me as far as the baby went not to have this baby in the hospital, and then somebody else just couldn't believe that I had it at home and not in the hospital because they'd be so scared of having it at home.

Do you want to end up?

Johnnie: Well, I don't have anything *new* to say about it. Just what Victoria's saying: it *does* depend on the surroundings. Okay, now you know me and I know you: the more relaxed you are, the better it is for you. In that case, I try to be as nice to everybody. Of course, I'm that way in everyday life [laughter], but when I get somebody here, I try to make it just as comfortable as I can. Then I be glad—just like she brought Marlena along. I was glad because I enjoy the company. We had a lot of fun.

Marlena: We sure did. She and I snickered a lot.

Do you ever have to send someone out of the room, if someone is in the room that is not helping?

Johnnie: If they want them to go out, you know, I send them out. Now I don't just let anybody come in the room nowhere. But just like her husband and a friend of hers she got already when she brought with her—yeah, they can be in there. Sometimes when they really get to bearin' down and that baby's comin', sometimes they want *everybody* to go. So in that case, I tell 'em. Other than that, no, I don't send 'em out.

Marlena: And that was what we had even discussed beforehand. I said, "If you want me to leave at any time, it's okay." That it would never be taken as an offensive thing. It was just the fact that that's what she needed. And that's who you're there to make comfortable.

Victoria: I didn't know how I was gonna feel either. I didn't know what was gonna happen. I didn't know if I was gonna start yellin' at people or what.

> *Interview with Mary Beth Chambers, March 1983*
>
> Mrs. Chambers is a seventy-seven-year-old black midwife from rural Florida. She became a midwife unwillingly when a seasoned local midwife, preparing to retire, saw Mrs. Chambers in a dream as her likely replacement. Years later, again involuntarily, she was surprised with a retirement ceremony—compliments of her county health department.

When did you start delivering babies?

I think it was '52.

How many years did you practice?

I think it was thirty-two. It might have been a little bit more than that.

Thirty-two years? Do you know how many babies you delivered?

They're all in here [she's thumbing through old papers].

Oh, those are all your records.

Excusin' the ones in Georgia. I delivered some in Georgia. All these are Florida babies.

Why did you retire?

I'm seventy-seven years old. And, you know, it's a certain amount of babies they want you to catch. 'Cause wadn't no retirement put on us as I know nothin' about.

You just volunteered?

No, I didn't volunteer. I had when they come in with it, when the nurse told me that she couldn't sign up for us anymore because me and Sister Barton, we had less babies, caught—delivered—less babies. So I wadn't goin' to act like I didn't like about it. I went on with it 'cause it didn't matter with me. I was wore out anyway.

Pretty soon you didn't have any babies to deliver?

See, some of 'em be in different [counties] where there'd be a lot of babies, and they delivered a heap of 'em. They come in with a big bunch of 'em. And then me and [Sister Barton] was about the oldest ones in there, too. We gettin' on up in age. I think that had somethin' to do with it. We'd been in there longer than anyone else. Now, this new stuff come in here after we was off; we weren't in that at all. That come in after this.

What was this certificate for, just to honor you?

Yeah, they had a little ol' get-together there in this place, and she had these. They had the governor to sign 'em, and that's what they give us.

When they did that, did you tell them you were going to retire, or did they tell you you were going to retire?

I ain't told 'em, no; I wasn't the one told 'em I was gonna retire. They just called it retirement, 'cause I don't know nothin' *'bout* no retirement. I thought as far as retirement is concerned, it'd be you know it when you get in it, don't ya? A certain age you retire? A certain time? That was never mentioned, nothin' like that. But, as I told you, she just tol' me. One day I went in there, I had somethin' or other before them, she said, "You about ready to retire?" I said, "Well, if I have to, I will." I just [left it kinda light]. Later on after then, when [it was] time to sign for your license again, she didn't tell me. I know me and Esther Barton in at the same time. We had been in there longer than any other of 'em: MacBride, Johnnie, Elizabeth, and all of 'em come in under us. Rosalind come in right about 'long with us, a little bit behind us, wadn't much different in me and her. But me and Esther been there; we were practicin' at the same time. And we was the oldest ones in there; the older ones was dead. Some of 'em suggested that's why. So I guess it is. I didn't even try to question to find out because if they wanted it like that, why, they could have it. And so many places they was cuttin' out the midwives anyhow. So I thought they wanted 'em out of G—— County, too. I had some people to talk to me and said they would go back. I said, "No, you [ain't gonna go back] for me. It's alright. It's alright."

So you never delivered any more babies?

I didn't. I don't deliver no babies. I haven't delivered a baby—that was in '80, and I haven't delivered a baby since, and I will not because I don't have no license. I don't want none now since I've been off that long.

I guess you could go back and get one any time you wanted now with the new law.

I imagine so, but it be so much I'd have to go through with to get started again, and now I think you'd have to know how to take blood pressure and all that kind of stuff. See, when we was goin', you go around with the midwife; that was startin' off about ten visits. Whenever she go out on a patient, she call you, and you go with her, watch her till you go to so many—around about ten. *Then* you call in the doctor, and he come. Now Dr. S—— was my doctor. He come out and check me a time or two. S'pose to come out five times and watch the delivery, and then while you can go in, and he'll even [carry a person into the clinic, too], and you can go in there and make your rounds. My midwife, even after I made my rounds, she still come back with me with one or two babies, just to see how I was doin'. I'd send for her, and she'd come. But she wouldn't do nothin'; she'd just come and sit and see how I was goin' to do, to see if I was still doin' like I was supposed to. At that time a patient had to go to the clinic. If they engaged you, and they hadn't attended a clinic or doctor, you wasn't supposed to wait on 'em. We didn't wait on 'em unless they okayed 'em. Now, I have been to patients where when I *get* there, sometime I wouldn't know. They'd call me, and sometime they'd be on the farm.

And they'd go to the boss man, and he called me to come out there. Well, I'd go. Now, the clinic would give 'em a little card where the midwife would *know* whether they had attended or not. And when I'd get there and question them, they wouldn't have nothin' to show. Then I'd have to go back to the boss man's house and call. I've done it several times. Mis' H—— was in the office at that time. I'd call back and tell her that the person's in labor and needs somebody to do somethin', but she don't have no card: what must I do? And sometime, most likely, they send a nurse out to come on and check her. And then sometime she said, "Well, go ahead." Mis' H—— come herself sometime. "I'll be out there as soon as—you say she can't wait?" I said, "No, she can't wait; she's right at the end of deliverin' the baby." Well, you couldn't just let somebody lay there like that, but you had to let somebody know what kinda shape you was in. And so, I got along pretty good with that. And then if you was sittin' at one a length of time and you make no progress—[the mother] still was havin' pain but still wadn't dilatin'—you'd check 'em. Still wadn't dilatin' at all, well, you know somethin' was wrong, and you'd have to take 'em to a doctor. And I've had to take some to the hospital, and they delivered the babies there 'cause it wouldn't be safe for 'em to deliver home. But now you got to know enough about it to know when to take one. So I didn't have any trouble; I never had any [mother or] baby to die on me. I've delivered twins one time—well, I delivered 'em more than one time, but I delivered two set of twins—and one *born* dead. But I called the doctor to okay it because if you have a mother or a baby die while you're deliverin', well, see, that goes on your record. You got to have somebody to okay it and tell whether it died through the struggle of being birthed or it was already dead 'fore it come. I never heard of havin' nothin' wrong with my record at all. I never was questioned about not doin' the rules that was supposed to be done. I always had it pretty clear because I always go and check with the nurses whenever I had a case that seemed like it was gonna be kinda complicated. I'd always check with them. If you wanted to help somebody that's goin' to be a midwife, you can call them in to sit in with you. I have called a new midwife right over in this community to come and sit in. That helps them 'cause you have a certain number to get. You can't just go out and start out. You got to get a certain number and then you got to get a doctor to okay it.

That's getting hard to do now.

Well, you can't do it now, 'cause the doctors don't wanta do it. And I wouldn't go back with it now, 'cause the doctors wouldn't—you can't hardly get a doctor now. They don't want to deliver no babies, and I don't think you find many midwife nurses, do you?

Well, that's starting up now. More women are wanting to do it the way you did it in their own home, but doctors are making it so hard on them that they choose the next best thing—to be a midwife in the hospital.

They makin' it hard on 'em. Before I was off, we went to Tallahassee once or twice to a meetin'. I think it was an Indian woman—she delivered all of her babies, her and her husband. And they was there talkin' about it. A lot of the people wouldn't want to go to the hospital, but since they cuttin' down on 'em, they got to go somewhere. Them got to be so [tight]. It used to be a lot of midwives in G—— County, but it's not but just two now unless some of the rest of 'em gonna go back. Other counties—take D—— County up there—that's why we delivered so many babies in Georgia, 'cross the line up there in my home. I used to go up there about as regular as I did down here 'cause wadn't no midwives 'cross the state line. That's just the way of it. Sometime it's kinda rough with ya, though, but sometime if you get a patient that's taken care of theirself—see, all women don't take care of themselves. They just go ham-scram, any kinda way about their health. Some of 'em weigh too much and just go to the doctor when they want to, won't be checked, just go every now and then. And then they expect the midwives to deliver the babies. Just an ordinary midwife couldn't do it because she wouldn't a had no more medical training than just deliverin' babies. If somethin' else goin' wrong inside of you, you wouldn't know, 'cause you not supposed to set your hands up nobody. You only *look*. When you wanta know how they dilatin', how things look, you have them to lay flat on their back and sit their legs up, and then you look, but you don't put your hands up there.

I think that's changed now, too. I think you can under the new law.

Well, it may be because they said these new ones, they want them to know how to take blood pressure and all that. That's why I know it wouldn't be no need for me. I'd almost have to go back to school. Somebody'd have to train me to get lined up with that. But some of the young ones what's comin' out now, they can learn as they comin' on. Well, that would be alright.

Or some of the young ones could show you how to use the new equipment, and you could teach them how to deliver the babies. This young midwife I brought along with me convinced Rosalind of that.

She told me she wadn't. She hadn't talk to me since she said the woman be out. I didn't know no woman been out there. Mis' S—— told me. But she had told me *befo'* then, when she heard about all this, she say, "I know I'm gonna give up, because I never learned all that; I'd have to go back to school. I just . . ."

By the time we left that day, she was pulling out her bag and she was excited about starting up again.

She might do it. She might go back at it, I don't know. But I don't have no idea of goin' back. I don't care about goin' back now because it might have been good that I come off. I be bothered with arthritis sometime. Sometime they having the baby—especially some of these younger ones—they don't want to go through with it, and yet they still don't want to go to the hospital or they don't have nothin' to go to the hospital with. And I think they think that *you* can stop the pains, but you can't stop 'em. You're not supposed to stop 'em, and midwives don't supposed to give anything at all. You got to know when one you see has too much, take her up and take her on to the doctor. You don't give no medicine. You use your own mother wit sense about that.

How old were you when they retired you?

Let's see, I must have been seventy-four; I'm seventy-seven now. That was in '80.

What happened at that ceremony?

Well, Miss M—— [county health nurse] was the one, and the doctor—I can't think of his name—he was there. They had all of the midwives in there, and they just had a talk and dinner, and then they asked me to say whatever I desired to say—a word or two. The doctor said a word; also Miss M——. And that was all.

What did you say?

Well, I thanked 'em for appreciating me enough to have the luncheon *with* me, and I let 'em know that I enjoyed workin' with them, and if it was the rule for me to retire at this time, well, I would accept it. But I let 'em know *definitely* that I didn't know any too much about it, and they never just said directly. 'Cause she the one that asked me; said she couldn't sign another license. Wouldn't be capable for her to sign another license. I think that that time I had delivered [only] about three or four babies [that year]. And so I put it to that, and then I heard after then, it was that and the age. But *she* didn't tell me.

Why would she say she couldn't sign another license?

Well, I reckon it wadn't enough babies; that's all I should know.

But she let Johnnie and some of them others continue.

Oh, yeah, they had caught enough, see? And then they wadn't as old as us.

That's what Mrs. Stephenson was talking about, saying she had to have so many babies. That's not true now.

See, some of 'em catches a lotta, lotta babies. You take MacBride. She's on that end down there where the white and the blacks all are, and they don't go to the hospital real fast. She catches a lotta white babies down that end. Alright, over in some areas, it be some babies, but since with the welfare helpin' these younger women go to the hospital now, I wadn't gonna run nobody down and ask them to let me wait on 'em. They was the ones supposed to come to *me,* not me go to them. Now, I have caught a right smart of 'em alright, but it went to goin' where I didn't catch so many, and so I guess that was the rule. You had to have so many; she didn't say how *many,* but I said that on account of I didn't have many.

You didn't know it was a rule until they told you?

No, I didn't know that.

So it was you and Esther Barton that day who were retired. And that left the four.

That left the four. Wadn't but six of 'em; that left four.

Did you feel very badly about having to retire?

Oh, no, I didn't feel bad at all. I just never did understand definitely altogether what it was about, but no more than that's what she said. But I didn't feel bad. I just didn't know retirement went like that. She the one knows. Now, this last one about credit—I understand they're not goin' to do what they used to do by the midwives. I reckon it might be a good thing that I'm off. 'Cause you really can go there [to the county clinic] if you had any problem about deliverin' a baby; you could go there and they would give you some information or tell you directly what to do. And if anything went wrong, well, see, then you'd let them know about it, and they know how to vouch for you. But these others [provisions of new law] you got to—I imagine you're gonna have to learn somethin' or other to do for yourself. 'Cause I understood that the clinic wouldn't be by you like it used to be.

So in case someone sued you if the baby or mother got ill?

Well, I think that's the way it goin' now.

But you once were protected by the health department?

Yeah, you could be protected, especially when they done attended the clinic and know about it. And if you know one wadn't attendin' the clinic, don't go irregardless of circumstance, don't go. And if the *law* have to send you, then *he'd* back you up. But you just don't go. I've had some boss mens have a bunch of folks on their place, and he'd send for me. Somebody out there, when I get there, they wouldn't have their card, and I'd contact them [the clinic]. Well, I was thinkin' all the time that they had went. [The boss man] said, "Well, what you think?" I said, "Well, she gonna need somebody to do somethin' right away, but I'm not supposed to do anything." He say, "Well, I'll go in there and check her out, and if you think she can make it to the hospital, I'll get a way to send y'all on over there." So I'd always go on to the hospital with 'em. And tell the nurse just how they reacted at home, and then let 'em be delivered there.

I heard them talking about these big bosses who would pay for the care. What's that all about?

Well, they'd be on a farm, see. A long time ago the people used to have these big tobacco farms, and it be plenty of people on there. As a rule, some people who do this don't look out for theirselves, none at all. And when that time come, well, they probably have a husband, a bunch of children workin' and all. The boss men, they *would* pay for 'em. They'd do that, I know. 'Cause I've got my money—I imagine, a heap a times, if the boss man didn't pay me, I wouldn't gotten none. He paid me, and then they'd have to pay him. Well, he paid them the money; he'd just take outta his money, and they'd get the rest. That's the way some of 'em be.

They'd mostly come for a midwife?

Yeah, that's mostly the way they would do. Now, some of 'em be on the farm and would do their own thing, but the common run of 'em, especially them that's old whiskey-heads, they wouldn't know. I've had some to come here at me so full until I couldn't hardly stand to go with 'em—see, I didn't drive at night. They'd have to come at me. If they wanta use me, they'd come at me. That's the way I started off, and that's the way I ended up. 'Cause I know Mis' M—— asked me on time, did I go? And I said, "No, ma'am, I don't drive at night." "Oh they come and get you." "Yes, ma'am, they come and get me; if they wanta use me, they come and get me. If they don't, well, I just stay home." That might be some reason why I didn't catch no more babies than I did.

Do you have any midwives in your family?

The midwives in my family dead. My great aunt, she was a midwife and a cousin, her daughter, was a midwife. I only had one child in my life, and that delivered *that* child for me. But both of 'em's dead.

Is that what made you want to go?

Well, I don't know. That didn't make me want to go, 'cause I was livin' down here a good while. But it was a lady named Eliza Overton. She's dead. That's the one I trained under. She delivered a baby in J——. She said she was wantin' to quit, and she had went to Dr. S—— and told him that she was gonna stop. She was old, and she was tired. He say, "Well, you got to get somebody." And she went to studyin' and prayin' and say I come before her one night. She had delivered a baby right in this community, down in the mine corp—when the mine was all abloom. And she come back to check the baby like we always do. When she come back, she sent for me to come down to the house where she was at. And when I went, she said, "Now, you who I wanta see." She said, "Friday, I want you to meet me in H—— and go to Q—— with me. I want to turn you in to the clinic. I want you to take my place." And I said, "Well, Eliza, I don't particularly want to be no midwife. I've been with the doctor at home. A white lady I used to work with, I was with the doctor with her. With all of hers, I was the midwife, but I just assist him." She had hers at home, you know, and

I'd be there with her. I say, "I don't wanta deliver no babies." She said, "Yeah, I want you to. I'm comin' on. Dr. S—— said I had to get somebody in my place. I pray to the Lord, and I saw you. You stood right before me, and I want you to take my place." She was a sweet old lady. I wouldn't deny her. I got up that mornin', got my husband to take me to H——. We caught the bus. When I got there, she was there. And we went on to Q—— to the clinic. So she turned me in and told the nurses she was gonna be with me until I make my rounds and get my license. And she did. When I went around ten times with her, then she called in Dr. S——. And Dr. S—— went 'round, I think, about three times. He okayed me, and he called in to the nurse and told Mis' H—— to give me my license, said that he was satisfied I knowed what to do 'cause I was under one of the best midwives that was, Eliza Overton. "I okay her," he said. "And if she need me, I'll go. I told her she get in a tight [situation] and need me, I'd go." And he did. He come to the last— until I got, you know, on the way.

So you didn't really want to be a midwife, but you couldn't say no to her?

I didn't particularly want to be one, but I did on account of her.

Did you do any praying about it?

No, I didn't pray about being one, but after I got to *be* one, then I shore did have to pray. 'Cause when I go on cases, you know, I want the Lord to go with me where I could have success. I'd asked him.

Did you start to like doing it?

I liked it pretty good while I was doing it. But sometime you'd get up and almost leave here in the storm. Somebody's in labor, and it's pouring down rain, oh, my Lord. I know I went to Georgia one night, and my husband in there, before he died, he said, "Well, you shore is crazy. I [bet ya before I'd get out from here], they'd take that woman and carry her on to the hospital or somewhere." But I went, and I've did that several times now. Talk about praying—but pray then because an old piece of car, it's dark on the road, you don't know when you're gonna run in the ditch or somethin' gonna run into ya. And you had to carry the Lord wit'cha. But I always had good success, good luck. I never had no problems.

What did you do while you were waiting with the mother? Talk?

Yes, just talk. Sometime I'd read. I had an Old Testament—sometime I'd read it. Try to cheer 'em up. Sometime some of 'em would, oh, just seem ready to go all to pieces. You'd try to tell them funny things, make 'em laugh. Sometime I'd get cool water and bathe their face off. Sometime I carry chewing gum or candy or somethin' that was in my pocket. I'd say, "Oh, I know, you just want a piece of chewing gum to chew on." Somethin' that'll just try to entertain her when you find one that's, oh, just don't wanta do *no* way. I delivered some women that didn't never take the snuff out their mouth. I don't see how they did that, but they did it, never took it out. I'd ask 'em, "Don't you want to rinse your mouth out?" "Mm-hmm."

So in a way, you had some kind of a calling through her.

Yeah.

What were you doing at the time?

I used to work over here on the W—— Farm. They'd come in the barn; I have to close out and go, just leave. I have left my food on the stove, turned it off and go. You have to go. Then sometime, you'd go, and if you'd knowed it before you left home, you woulda had time to stay home and finish doin' what you was doin'. But you don't know until you get there. And I have went and come back and went back again. But now you got to be sure 'cause some of 'em are in a slow labor, and, boy, every now and then, they'll make a contraction. You don't wanta just sit there all day and all night and just get tired and wore out. So I left and come back. Sometime I have left, at home, and probably stayed a couple of hours, and come back. They've picked up and goin' right on at it. When I get there, I wouldn't have a thing to do but wash my things, 'cause everything you carry will be sterilized and put up. I just put my things out and get ready. Put the leggin's on them and put the—sterilate them across the stomach.

Did you have to shave them?

Yes, you had to shave them. And later on they come about with the shave proposition, and you do that. And after you clean 'em up down there, then you just sit there and watch until the water bag push out. You tell 'em when to push, not in a strainin' way, 'cause some of 'em'll start the pushin' [by the] time a little stingin' pain hits 'em, and that just gives 'em out. You're not suppose to do like that. But you probably can get 'em to understand just exactly what to do and when.

You never delivered babies at your home?

No, ma'am, I never delivered none. I didn't want that job. I wadn't gonna fix no place to deliver no babies on. I go to they home.

Why didn't you want to do it at home?

Why I didn't want one? I just didn't want one. I thought that anyone who wanted a baby oughta . . . [Laughter.] I'd had to work and build another room and all, and it wasn't worth all that 'cause sometimes, in some cases, you have a time gettin' your money.

How much were they charging then?

Well, when I come off, it was fifty dollars. But I think it's more now.

I think it's up to a hundred twenty-five dollars now. I think they're letting people charge whatever they want.

This new thing, I think, is they're not pacin' it no more.

How many times would you go back and see the mother after the baby was born?

In generally, two times. Sometimes we make the third time, 'cause sometimes little complications arise, and they send for ya. Some of 'em get up a little faster than they ought to do, and you go back and check 'em over again and see whether they need to go to the doctor. But in generally, I didn't have any trouble much. We'd have to go back once or twice 'cause the baby's navel had to be looked at. You wouldn't want just anybody to do it—not while it was like that before it get well—'cause a lot of times the people don't have their hands good and clean, and they're messin' around in there and get germs in it, and that'll upset it. You want to attend to it yourself until it get kinda well where you could turn it loose. We always had a ruler, used little Scotch pads, Scotch drawers, and leave a few of 'em there. The mother could put them on if she wanted or use sterile gauze. This little Scotch soft cloth is good, [but] they stopped using it. They didn't demand us to use that, but that's a good way to heal 'em up. Then they just have to put a clean gauze on it.

When you delivered babies, was it mostly just you and a mother, or were there other people in the room?

Well, sometime you have to ask some of 'em out. Sometime there be a little bit *too* many. But you like for somebody to be in there with you, 'cause after you start with her, you wouldn't want to take your hands offa her and go put on anything; you have somebody to hand you different things that you wanted to use, like little basins and whatnot.

What did everybody else do?

Other people be sittin' there lookin' till you get 'em out the room. I always get 'em out. I didn't like a room full. The mother and somebody else is enough for me.

Did you have any fathers stay in the room?

The fathers could stay in there if they wanted to, but hardly ever you'd find a father. Every now and then he'd stick his head in the door, say, "Everything alright?" They'd ask the question, but they wadn't particular about stayin' in.

So it'd usually be the woman's mother?

Yeah, her mother or sister. Sometime, some of 'em have a friend of theirs to stay in the room.

Were these usually women who'd had babies before?

Yeah, most likely. 'Cause them that never had none, they'd be more hollerin' in the room than you would want. You wouldn't need them in there. They make it tough. [Laughter.] Yeah, you didn't need them in there at all. 'Cause somebody already been through it, well, they understand. And they wouldn't be near as bad.

What do you remember about those midwives that came before you? What kind of women were they? Were they church women? Was the midwife someone everyone knew in the community?

Oh, yeah. The one that I come up under, she was a religious lady. And there was another one, Sheila Harry, that's the one Rosalind Stephenson come up under. Uh-huh. She lived down the highway there. She was a fine person, too. I remember when she died. And when Eliza died. And there was another one, Lucy Wilson, stayed up the highway from Q——. She died. And Susan Bradley, she was a old lady. She died, too. In fact, all the older ones died out, as I said. Esther and me was the next oldest ones. The others had died. They all was religious people. They all was. And Elizabeth's mother, Annie Black, and her sister Martha Graham, they all died. All of 'em was religious people.

Have you delivered a lot of babies from one family?

Well, that house right there [points out the window to house across clay road], I delivered all that girl's children except three—the three oldest ones. I wadn't deliverin' then. I think she was the one that I went to see this lady about, to the house where this woman [Eliza Overton] had dreamt for me to come, when she come back to see the girl. All the rest of her children, I delivered 'em. There's Ellen, Bonnie, Sherrie, Candace—I think it's five. And it's several homes where they older ones was [born] mostly before I started. I got several families like that. This woman that works in the clinic over there in Q——, I delivered all of hers but three. Dr. M——, I think, delivered hers in his lifetime 'cause he delivered a lot of babies. After I got to be a midwife, I delivered all of hers. And they was all over there, right across the creek over there on the W—— Farm. There's several homes that, when I become a midwife, I delivered the rest of their babies.

But when you get a midwife, you usually stick with the same one.

Yeah, they wouldn't hardly change.

Did you ever deliver a mother and daughter?

Yes, I delivered a mother and daughter, and they're right there [same house across road]. And they was kinda close together. The daughter had hers a little ahead of the mother. And both of 'em is outta high school. I think they're goin' to the technical school in T——.

What do you think the future for the young midwives in T—— will be?

I don't know. Is really some tryin' to do it? Well, they probably will do alright if they go to workin' and learn all these other things they want 'em to do, they'll do alright. I imagine it'll be good for 'em. But I declare, some of the poor people, I declare, I don't know how in the world they get to the hospital; it's so high just ordinarily, if there ain't nothin' the matter. I can see if you're sick and they got to do something for ya, but just normal baby deliverin' . . .

There are some young white women in T—— who want midwives not just because of the high price of the hospital but because they just want to do it at home. So that's why all this legal fighting started. Do you want to add anything we might have left out?

Well, I don't know anything particular pertainin' so directly to that. While I was deliverin' babies, I just tried to do my best that was in my power to comfort the mothers. I'd pay strict attention to the action of 'em so if they needed help that I couldn't give, I would move in time to give 'em the right help. I was just like that about it 'cause I didn't want nobody to suffer. I know to have your baby, you got to go through with *somethin';* it's not gonna be all that easy all the time, and it ain't gonna be as hard as some think. But the thing of it is, if you be one, why, the learnin' enough about the person to see just when she's sufferin' too much without help—that was the main thing. And I studied that harder than I did anything else. I really did because I didn't want to lose a patient. I didn't want that on my record nowhere. And you have to study it, too, 'cause you have to *know* when to make the move when one couldn't be at home. 'Cause if you didn't pay 'em much attention, something seriously might happen, and when you would take a notion to look, it be too late.

How did you get to know them? Did you do prenatals then?

Yes, you go to see 'em when they engage ya. They supposed to engage ya. You didn't have to go if you wadn't engaged unless it was a bad case of emergency. I mostly went and checked with my head nurse. Right about three months, they supposed to engage you. When they go to the clinic, the clinic gonna ask them, "Who gonna deliver your baby?" And they gonna give them the name of that person. The nurse at the clinic will have to get in contact with you and let you know that so-and-so is dependin' on you to deliver their baby, and they're takin' the treatments alright. It'd be alright for you to go. Now they gonna do that. Now, where one don't tend, you go every now and then, and they don't have no proof of records or nothin', they don't urge you to go. They have to have somethin' or 'nother. You don't have to just go unless you want to. That's why I said a while back, sometime some of the farmers—some of the bosses—they would have [inaudible], and the clinic wouldn't have much of a record on 'em, but when they go get confined and that [husband] probably been drunk all the weekend or somethin' or other, he'd run up there to the boss and say his wife was in labor and she had to have a midwife. The boss said, "Well, who do you want?" He'd give 'em my name. "Take the car. Go get her." And then when they get there and check 'em out and things ain't right, then you got to let somebody know about it. I had one boss man, he was very good. I'd go to him and explain the situation to him. 'Cause if one of 'em on his place, I didn't even undo my bag. I said, "I'm not gonna undo my bag. You take her to the hospital." He took her. That's right, he shore did. He said, "Well, you go along with her, and I'll have 'em to bring you back. I'll call over there and tell 'em to take care." And I went on with her to try to cheer her up, make her feel good goin' home. We carried her on to the emergency room, and they checked her out. Some of 'em come out pretty good. I have delivered ones.

Is it that hard to deliver breech babies?

All the time; it's not easy.

Now they don't even fool with it if it's breech; they do a C-section.

Well, sometime the hips are out, but now the arms can be stretched this way. You see, that's not right. Now, if they right down side of her, it come out easy. But if they stretched inside of you, it's gonna upset somethin' and probably have an infection or somethin' and you gonna need somebody. So if you see one in time, you take 'em somewhere else where they had the equipment, things you can do it with. At that time, we wadn't puttin' no hands inside nobody. And you couldn't help 'em with the baby comin' like that. 'Cause if the hands was inside, it wadn't no way for you to help them unless you could've put yours in there and then pull it down, but then you probably would've been tearing something else a-loose. It wouldn't be safe to do that, and none of us didn't try it. I'm quite sure none didn't, 'cause I know I ain't never tried it. I never heard nobody else tryin' it. Now, I have delivered a breech 'un, but he was comin' so fast, there was no other way for him to do but to let him come on, but he come straight. All of 'em don't be straight. If they come straight, it's alright. When I see the feet comin' first, all I was anxious about seein' was the head.

Can you keep that from happening? How does the baby turn around?

I don't know of no way of disposition. I don't know what causes a baby to be in that disposition. But that's why if they took an examination regular like they should, they would know. But see, half of 'em don't.

But at the last minute the baby can turn around?

Yeah, it turns around more likely. 'Cause all of 'em don't be sittin' there right. You can feel the stomach and feel he's sittin' right straight up. But the time for that baby to come, nature turns the head down. That's why I like to see the head. But he gonna make a turn; if he's sittin' in a position for him to make this turn when the head come down, it's comin' down. And if he's in the other position, when he make that turn and his butt's comin' down, it's gonna come down. But I always like the head. The safest way.

*   *   *   *   *

I think the doctors don't care anything about deliverin' no babies. They didn't want some nurse-midwives in the hospital. I don't think they want 'em, but they would. They could do it 'cause the doctors didn't care about it. I didn't have too much trouble. The years I was [practicing], I think it was pretty good. I never been in real close cor-

ners, not really. Maybe one or two little problems. It didn't take me
long to get right quick to where I could get help. So it come out alright.
I wasn't slow enough to keep somebody home and let something bad
happen to 'em. I always tried to stay on the alert in time enough to get
'em away.

How long has that hospital been there?

Oh, I believe that hospital was put there in '52, 'cause I went there in
'52 for an operation—it just had been built.

So there used to be no hospital around here before that.

No, doctors had to come to your house. We had a doctor up here
on the edge of Georgia, Dr. M——. I've called him, and in H——, Dr.
S——. I've called him. I think those others on the other side, Dr.
B—— and them, were before the hospital got [built]. But if you had to
have a doctor, you'd get somebody to come.

Did midwives do a lot of other healing?

I don't know about the real old ones, but along in my time, when I
started, it wasn't all that much that you did. Now all the real old wom-
en's done gone.

Interview with Mary Keller, August 6, 1981

Mrs. Keller is a very old black woman from north Florida who had all her babies with the same midwife.

How many children did you have?

Well, I'll tell you. I had four. I had a boy, and I had three girls. There's two died.

How did they die?

They was sick.

But they died after they were born?

Oh, they were grown, was out and married. And I had two or three grandchildren. And they grown now.

Well, I just want to hear you tell me about your childbirths at home with a midwife or other women present.

Oh, in them days there was women—wasn't no doctor . . .

Right, that's what I'm interested in.

Oh, about the old folks, the old midwives. She's dead now, *been* dead, and she come and did for us when I was having my baby. But in them times they didn't have what they got now at the hospital. You had a nurse, a midwife—they call it midwife. I had that baby, and she come and wait on me, and I couldn't get out to eat nothin'—just stay there till the time for me to get out under what she doing for me.

She cooked for you and fed you?

No, my mother. They see to me and feed me. She'd tell her what to give me, you know. I have been where I couldn't get nowhere. I couldn't go outdoors about two or three days. I had to stay in the house with a little something or other on his head, a little cap.

[Laughter.] You remember? I don't know, you don't know nothing about that. I couldn't move out until that hour for me to get out from having this baby. And I go out, and I be scared myself 'cause I didn't know where it was gonna do anything. And she'll come back; the nurse will come back and let me know when to go out.

You mean the midwife?

Yeah. They'll come out and let you know what time you can get out on the ground with your baby.

When you had the baby—do you remember your first birth? Who else was there besides the midwife?

Oh, nobody. I ain't never had none with no doctor here. I had *midwives* in them days. Wadn't no doctor. There was a doctor, but we always wanted a midwife. But she's dead now.

You had the same one every time?

Yeah, the same one.

Did she deliver you from your mother?

No, ma'am, it was *my* babies.

You remember the first birth?

I had a boy.

Did she stay with you?

No, she go home.

When you were having the baby, though, did she—

She stayed right there till he come.

Did she read the Bible to you?

No, she didn't read no Bible. 'Cause she just stay there, and she'll catch that baby and wash him off and put him back in the bed there with me.

If you had to do it today—if you could have a baby today—

No! No! [Laughter.] I wouldn't.

—would you have it in the hospital or would you have it at home like the way you had it?

I would like to have it at home, 'cause if I had a nurse, they know what to do 'cause they done went to the doctor, and the doctor told them. They went through all that for how to take care of babies. I never had any child in no hospital. I always had it at the house till the midwife come—in them days they didn't have no doctor. Doctor didn't have to go do *nothin'*. I reckon sometimes he tells them what to do, but he didn't tell us. The nurse would come and tell us. We couldn't eat nothin' till *she* tell us to eat. We have certain foods to eat when they get that baby. She ain't going to let you eat everything. She'll tell you what to eat and drink a little milk. And you don't eat everything, 'cause you see, you got to wait till that baby get a little certain age to eat anything heavy like it ain't fittin'. You have to eat what she tell you, and you know you be so hungry when the time to eat. [Laughter.] You don't have nothin' to eat 'cause when you do it, you eat too much when you ever start. And she took care of that baby; we couldn't pick 'em up. She comes every time and wash him. [Laughter.] And she wash him and put him back, and they give you little bottle, you know, with milk in it just to let them suck.

Did you breast-feed your baby?

Yeah, after I got well, I sure did feed them. I just take my breast, one of them, and pull it out and let them nurse the best way they could.

What do you think of women who have stopped breast-feeding?

Well, I don't think they're right, because look like they *should* go back in the old way of doin'. But a heap of 'em don't. You get out and the next morning they can come out anywhere of the hospital. But you got to stay in there several weeks 'fore you get out; the midwives ain't going to turn you loose, 'cause they think you catch cold. Remember? And so we had to stay in there until that time came to get out. Until *she* tell you that it's time.

Your mother didn't come in while you were having the baby?

No, she don't come in there. She could hear that baby cry, but she can't come until the nurse *tell* her to come.

What do you think about people who have the father in the room?

Well, I ain't never had that, with the father come in the room.

Did you have an easy first birth?

No, Lord! It was hard. I never had it before, but I said I always didn't want me another one, but I did get another one after that. Oh,

I'm telling you, it's a hard job when you having a baby. And I'm telling you, and I already don't want me another one. I had about five children; so I just knocked off. I ain't had no more. I got those with the midwives. It ain't like it is now. I ain't never had no baby for them like the doctors. I had 'em for midwives because midwives come to see you all the time. Now, she might miss this morning; she'll come and find out how you getting along before you have the baby. And she would tell you what to eat and what not to eat.

Once you start going into labor, she'd stay with you right up to the end?

Yes, she stay there till it's all over with. Sometime it ain't all over till maybe the first day when you get that pains. But by the next day, she might come and see how you're doing. And she know what time the baby going to come. She know the hour. Mm-hmm.

How does she know that?

I don't know how she know it, but she'll know it. That's a hard thing to bring when you got one coming. Yes, it's a hard way to bring babies like that, without a doctor.

Think a doctor would make it easier?

I don't know. I ain't never had none by a doctor, only had midwives. And all them days they just stopped the midwives, and then [women started] going to the doctor.

Do you think it is good or bad that the midwives are dying out?

I would rather have the midwives 'cause they always come and see about you, to see how you're doing before you ever have the baby.

They'll sit down and talk to you how to do and not to eat. And that's all? That's all was going with no doctors, 'cause they never come in them days. Nothin' but midwives. And they just cut off all those midwives. There no midwives to wait on nobody that I think about. Ain't never hear talk of none. But I believe they should go back and *get* those midwives. 'Cause they comes and sees about ya 'fore you ever have the baby.

When you have the baby, do you feel any spiritual feelings about it?

No, you feel like you done got the load off you when you have the baby. And you just lay there and eat what they tell you to eat till the time come for you to be out. But now they mostly let you outta the hospital as soon as the baby born. One time, my daughter—after she got married—she had a child, and I went up there to the hospital to see her, and she was eating something like that. I say, "Why did you eat this? Ain't this bad?" She said, "The doctor told me to eat it." I say, "I wouldn't never ate it 'cause I didn't ever eat it, and now here you're eating it. A piece of chicken."

How long did you have to wait before the midwives would let you eat?

I don't know exactly how long, but I know they didn't allow you to eat all kinds of things. She was sitting up there eating chicken and everything. I say, "You eating chicken here, and you just now had your baby." She say, "Well, he told me." I said, "Well, we didn't ever do that." But they didn't take it like I did. They leave out the place look like before they should leave out to be walkin' around. We didn't do that. We had to have a certain hour. Same time for to come out. If us did come down, they'd say, "Why y'all doin' what you're doin'? You ain't supposed to come out here before your time to get up and walk." But these people's time, they go to the hospital and have the baby;

about two or three days, they out and eating everything. And I know I couldn't do it. I was scared to eat things, 'cause they come and tell you what to eat, those old midwives. I liked the midwives better than I do in the hospital.

Interview with Mary Lee Jones, April 28, 1984

> Mrs. Jones is a seventy-nine-year-old black urban midwife from Florida. She operated a maternity home and claims that her trade was passed down through her family and given to her by God. In addition to delivering over five hundred babies, she delivered herself of three of her own children, unassisted.

The only thing I know about you so far is that you feel you had some kind of calling.

Mine come from God.

Tell me about the beginning—how you got into it, how old you were.

Well, I always want it from a little girl. If I saw a lady pregnant, if Mama didn't watch me, I'd follow as long as I could see her. 'Cause I *loved* it! And once, I guess I was about nine or ten, they had a lady to have a baby. Well, they wadn't gonna let me in. So I went under the house. I was interested—from that instant [pounds table], it was all my life; I wanted to be a midwife.

You were in the room when the baby was born?

No, I didn't get to go in; I was under the house! I went under the house.

Could you hear what was happening from under the house?

No, I just thought I would hear something. But I heard the baby cry. That was the only thing that I could hear, but I didn't hear anything else.

So you didn't become a midwife till you were how old?

Mmm, thirty somethin'. Well, in this county, I was on 1940, and I'm seventy-nine now.

Let's see, you were thirty-nine when you started?

You see, I was workin' before I was licensed because I'd been workin' with doctors. I would say I was in my early thirties.

After your babies were gone?

No, I delivered right along with mine. And I delivered three of my *own*. All boys; I didn't have but one girl. All the rest of 'em boys; I delivered three of them. Really, I *loved* it, and I thought if I could wait on somebody else, I could do it for myself.

Tell me about your midwife relatives.

My grandmother a midwife; my aunt was a midwife, and my mother. I've been trying to get some of my *grand*children. I tried to get my daughter; she said, "No, girl!" She wouldn't do that! [Laughter.]

Why not?

She didn't like it. But I did; I just wish I could deliver one about every day. I just *love* it! But, you know, it's out. I mean, they didn't take

my license or nothin'. I just had to stop. They put so much pressure o
us. See, when we get a certain age, you done learn to live with a littl
pressure.

How'd they do that?

They want me to go back to school. You know, I can't go back to n
school just like that 'cause that's too much on me. I delivered all thos
children, and I delivered less than fifty years in O—— County. An
before I came to this county, I delivered in Georgia; I was workin' wit
the doctor. Well, if he didn't get there in time, the baby come. I didn'
leave; I stayed.

*Did you have to have referral cards from the health department? Di
they have to get their prenatals at the department of health?*

Not at the health department, but some doctor. A long time ago, th
ladies didn't go to the doctor. That doesn't count now, you know; the
got along just as well, but we can't change the law. That's right, w
can't change it no way. Women didn't have to go, and we didn't hav
no trouble.

But the law changed your whole tradition.

Right. So many things they are changing they shouldn't change
Even the sun—I mean, the time. I don't like it; I just think they shoul
let it stay . . .

Why do you think they changed all that?

Modern times makes a mess of a whole lot of things. [Laughter.] It
nice to be modern. A lot of things now, so many was uncalled for. W

got along very well. Anybody that was gonna have a baby, and they heard about me, they'd come get me any time o' night, anything. But no doctor hadn't seen them 'cause most of 'em didn't have any money. I didn't worry about money if the Lord had blessed me to help somebody; I've always gone. But I didn't worry about it—I *still* don't worry about it.

Tell me more about your calling; how did God want you to be a midwife?

Well, I guess it's come from the beginning of it, because my aunt, I trained under her awhile. When she passed, I got all her equipment. I wrote to Jacksonville for the license, and they wrote me back a letter, told me they had enough midwives. But I didn't stop. I wrote 'em right back and told 'em my aunt was dead, that she give me everything, she wanted me to take her place, and they sent me the license.

Your aunt told you that before she died—that she wanted you to take over?

Oh, yes.

Seems like a lot of midwives want somebody to carry on after them.

Just like me. I'd be tickled to death. I had a letter from one lady in Jacksonville; the lady wanted me to *train* some midwives, such as *I* know. I wanted to do it, and I have asked for permission; I'm gonna try it. And anyone who want to come up, they can come on under me. Now, if they object, they say you just can't do it—that's all. I don't see nothin' wrong with it.

Recently they asked you to train?

Yeah, last year. When I first started, I had to go out—we were out there working *with* the doctor. I had to go out with the doctor fifteen cases before they would issue my license. And I got it.

Think that was about right or too much?

That was too much. But I don't know, 'cause I wanted the job, and I was willing to sacrifice anything in the world that I could do to get it.

So how big was your practice at one time?

Well, oh, well, I had a *big* practice.

Here or in Georgia? I saw you were from Georgia.

Yeah, but I was working with the doctor. I was licensed in 1932 right here in O—— County.

How many were you delivering on the average?

Well, I have delivered eighteen babies in a month. Eighteen babies in one month! And the nurses was on then, and they would say, "Well, you won't do that again." And I don't know if they meant it like—I don't know. It made me feel bad. But that's what they say. *Eighteen* babies! I was *workin'* that month. *Never* home!

Did you go to their house?

Oh, yeah!

Did you have any here?

Yes, I used to run a maternity place over at that house over there [points to the house next door].

Was this house standing here?

Yeah, I had moved here.

So you operated a maternity home, and you lived over here?

Mm-hmm. I lived over there with 'em mostly. I just love my work, and I wanted to see what's happenin'.

Well, what happened with that?

They started complainin'.

Who complained?

The county. But I've had nurses—I've had doctors come out here— they'd deliver 'em out there. But I don't know, those complaints, I got discouraged . . .

What kind of complaints? Inspections and things? Code enforcement?

Well, I'll tell you, one inspector came out here once, and he didn't find nothin'. We weren't quite competing then, and he thought it was a great thing to have. But you know, what *he* feel back then [was an exception: there's so many others don't think you should].

So then you eventually just had to close down . . .

Well, the reason why I closed, my work begin to fall down. See wadn't no need to holdin' it with the little work I was gettin' to do. But a lot of time, I just continued going out to deliver. Babies wadn't as plentiful the last five or six years from then. Oh, but when there was plenty of babies, you get you a midwife. The doctors complain, but they had more work than they can do, more than they can takes care

So the complaints came from the doctors?

Yeah, the doctors, the nurses. Because some of the nurses [said] "Now you tell me, you just done got *that* low to have a midwife.' That's discouraging the lady. "Well, suppose so-and-so's gonna happen?" Nothin's gonna happen! If you put your trust in God, if anything happen, you know what to do. I never let one suffer yet.

Did you have any mothers die on you?

No.

A few babies?

Not many. I was *way* back there in the thirties—once in a while. That's like if I have a baby was born right there [the house next door], as soon as that baby's born, I got to call the health department. But they never did find anything wrong. [They'd go right through shortly after my deliveries.] We tried to do the right thing. I always have to [live] in the Lord. I do that now. Now, let me ask you something and see if you think it'd hurt me: you reckon they would object if some women's husbands wants to deliver the baby and want me to just come out and tell him *what* to do and what *not* to do? That's what I've been thinking about.

You mean coaching husbands?

Yeah, teach 'em what *I* know. Some men really wanted to when I was working. There's a lot of men be right there with me. Sure was. I have some men on the job, just before the baby born, they give out. [Laughter.] They couldn't take it. But most of 'em brave men.

I don't know, can you do that legally?

I don't know. I'm so afraid if I ask, they'll say no.

See, that's the thing, they're so afraid of being sued for malpractice.

Oh, idn't that the truth. 'Cause that's one reason why I was goin' to give up my license, because if anything they want to do, I would have to be responsible for the mother and the baby and anything else, and I don't have nothin' but this old house. To take that out of . . .

You don't own that house next door any more?

Yes, I still own it. After I stopped using it, then I had a home for old people.

You want to do that or you've done it?

I'm too old now, darlin'.

Now what do you do with it?

I rent it.

You know, there's so many women around the state like you; and it's really unfair.

And I wish, someday, that many of us could get together and meet in some place, and we could have a talk.

You need to organize.

That's what we need, but I wonder how we go about it. I've been thinkin' about it. A long time ago, way back, we used to have a state-wide convention, and the midwives come all over the state right here. Oooh! We had an awful good time!

Are you the only one left?

I'm the oldest one in this county—the only one left. And when I come on in '32, there was five hundred midwives in the state of Florida. I just pray—that's all we can do now. But if God don't take over, there ain't gonna be nothin' that's done because they don't *try* to do nothin' [more] to help the poor man than that—give us money, money, money. I mean, there's more to life than money. They need more love—that's the worst of all. 'Cause I've gone behind doctors and nurses that just didn't care. But if you had money, okay, I'd wait on ya, but if ya didn't have it, I would wait on you. 'Cause I [love 'em], and I knew just what they were goin' through. And they *need* somebody to have a baby. Money or no money, you got to have a baby.

Who did you apprentice under?

Oh, Dr. D——.

So you didn't go under another midwife? You went with your aunt, didn't you?

Not then. [I worked with my aunt], and then I worked with this doctor quite a lot.

To get your fifteen cases?

Yeah. And then if I got into any trouble anywhere, night or day, he'd come to my call. I had lots of 'em, a lot of times it was here, and I had to call. I mean all time of night, anything—he'd come see about ya. But you call now and see if you don't [die 'fore he get here]. [Laughter.] I love it, though. Only thing, if it just wadn't for this suing proposition, I think I woulda gone on through. But you never know. When you get up in years, somethin' like that, it makes you a little bit fearful. 'Cause you just don't know what may happen, and it's not good for ya.

The thing is, most parents who come to a midwife are the kind of people willing to take responsibility for their own birth and are not likely to sue.

Oh, yeah, yeah. But you know, in California, the family didn't sue that lady, but the *county* sued her. You remember that, don't you? These doctors been [bein'] themselves because Dr. W——, he know all about us. We were on with Dr. A—— for the last two or three years. He's a young doctor; when I'd send my patients, he'd [ask me].

What did he do?

Send them to the hospital.

And you thought that he was going to send them back to you?

Yes. See, I didn't know myself if I'm gonna work with the patient. They tell me, and I don't know. I guess I shouldn't have mentioned his name, but it's too late now.

I won't use it. So the thing is that people come back and tell you they can't have the baby with you because the doctor said they had something that meant they needed to be in the hospital?

Yeah, so many times, they would tell them different things. "Well, you have so-an'-so; you better have it at the hospital." And then the womens get frightened—they are scared.

Then, by the time you have all your prenatals with someone, I guess you figure you'll go ahead and have the baby with them, too. They're sneaky.

You ain't kiddin'. That's right. Well, I have one or two black women, one or two white women, wants to become a midwife, but I just don't know whether they goin' to accept 'em; they gonna put 'em through a lot of red tape, I can tell 'em that. You got to have grits if they want to come, they're not gonna let 'em turn 'em down.

They want to apprentice under you?

Yeah, they just wanta let me tell 'em. I don't mind tellin' 'em. I let 'em come over here [and] I'll teach 'em everything that I've done. I don't know whether it's gonna work, but I'm gonna try. I might begin with this girl out here, with this lady in Jacksonville.

I think that's a good idea. It's a good use you can put your skills to. And if nothing else, you get to be at births again.

It's kinda hard; but I don't care, I love it.

What kinds of things did you do during birth; what was your bed-side manner like?

Just any little thing. If we wanted to clean the house up, we'd cook or clean up. If us ever was needed for this, we would do that. Sometime they'd go to have the babies, just wouldn't have nothin' prepared; we'd make somethin' the babies put on—we *all* did things like that. 'Cause I just enjoyed it so much. Everybody don't be prepared. A long time ago, we didn't use anything but newspapers.

Did they make you start shaving the women, too?

They'd make you do it, but so many of 'em I didn't shave. If they didn't want it, I didn't shave 'em. They can't *make* you shave 'em; there's no law for that. 'Cause I never was shaved for any of *my* children.

Well, they're finding now that shaving—when it breaks the skin—if there's any infection it will get to the bloodstream.

But what about the doctors when they cut 'em? What's the difference? I don't know, most people don't like it. Then if they just don't like it, I cut it as low as I can get it. That's a help, [but lots] of that blood stuff, you know, it comes over there sometime. I did everything I could.

Did you have to do episiotomies?

No, no, the doctors do that.

But you never had women tear?

Well, yes, a little bit, but I worked with the doctor. He say if they done tear, just clean it. But it doesn't matter.

It heals?

It heals. There's a doctor right here in O—— that say as long as you don't cut, they don't need to put no stitches in there. Quite naturally, it will heal. It may depend on maybe if it didn't tear right. I 'magine if it crossed here like that, it might be a bit—I don't care how it's torn. They gonna heal back 'cause they all together down there.

I have found some minutes to a meeting in which the same doctor who states that the midwives' statistics are better than the doctors' goes on to still refer to the "midwife problem" and phasing them out.

Well, I heard one doctor where he said, "It's better for a woman to have a baby at home than go to the hospital 'cause there's not as many germs in the home as there is in the hospital. They got all kind o' germs. He talk so good; I could have listened to him till . . .

Who's that?

A doctor was talkin' on the news. But I'll take a chance if we get over this suing proposition, 'cause you don't know never when they get there and you be ruined. And I don't have anything. What I have I need 'cause I'm too old to get anything else. I been years and years gettin' this little house, and I'm gonna keep it. Now, when I moved in 1949, my children was in college, in different places, wadn't [no one] but myself and my husband. So that made a big gap in a big house.

You really long for it.

Oooh, I *love* it! And now, you know, they wanted me to deliver that baby on [a nationally syndicated television news program]. And look like the thing [lay midwifery] ain't goin' back 'cause they didn't want me to pay for my license.

They came after you when they saw you on television?

Yes, ma'am. See, then they wanted me to pay for my license. But all these many years, I never had to. The state always give me my license [but the county had been cruel]. But I never didn't have no trouble—never, never!

So you were the last midwife around here for a long time? Were they still having those monthly midwife meetings?

Oh, no, years and years they ain't had one. But I used to have to go to the clinic; they used to have a meeting every Monday at the clinic. And we'd have to go to this meeting with more than myself. But if it come down to me, they'd forgot I was out there, and they was glad when I was gone. [Laughter.]

The women in G—— County are still practicing.

Oh, yeah? Oh, good. Well, I've had to deliver a baby out of this county. But I've had some in P——, and all down there they couldn't afford a doctor. But they didn't know what happened. The nurse told me that I couldn't take nothin' none from W——, but I had a nice lady over in W——. She said you can't go out to practice . . .

But you'd go anyway?

[Laughter.] I went in there with the Lord because I don't give up, and the people was so nice that I couldn't give it up. You've got to [avenge 'em]. They won't let you deliver to keep your practice. And all this fighting education—I just think that's wrong the way they fightin' education. Now, I was promoted to the fourth grade. I didn't study, and I'll put myself up with any doctor—I don't care who he is. If he just use his head, I'd deliver a baby as quick as he could. But see, you [can't go now with the old stuff]. I mean, my aunt didn't know a *a* from a *b*. She didn't know a thing—no education. What little I had I just kept adding to; I just kept lovin' and studyin' my job, and I got alright. You gotta have experience and nerves and everything else when these people [get to hangin' on].

Don't you think you have to be a certain kind of person? Not just anybody can be a midwife. That's why I think there's something to this idea of being called to it.

Yeah, I was called from God, and I delivered 'em all 'cause when they started talkin' about it, I tell 'em [even then before I was called]. When they issued me the license, God gave me the job. And I sure hate—

To be apart from something you want to do?

That's right. So I'm just around. But I'm glad to do anything I can to help the next person who want to come on—*glad to.*

Why do you feel so strongly about getting one of your own relatives?

They won't accept it.

But why do you feel like you'd really like one of your children to carry on your practice?

I have two little granddaughters. I have a little granddaughter in T—— in college now, but she won't—she don't say she won't. She wants to see a baby born. Maybe if I could get her to see one born, I hope I can get her to take the trade. Because I asked her a couple years ago when she's finishing, I said, "Why don't you take up midwifery on the side? That would be a help to [me]." But these young people, I don't know . . .

She doesn't want to do that?

I don't think so. Now, I have another one in T—— now—oh, no, she's home right now. And she told me when she finishes up that she was gonna take it. But I don't know if she's gonna take it.

What was she training in up there?

I don't know.

Nursing?

No, not nursing. Nah, I don't know whether she'll be able to. They want you to get in nursing. She might be a nurse-midwife, but you know, that's uncalled for. And they charge so much money. Why I don't know. I know people have to have money; they want it to do other things with it, but God take a person that doesn't have and give 'em a chance. Things gettin' to be bad with everything.

What was the old midwives' standing in the community?

Most people loved 'em. Now a lot of them say they just wished I was workin'. I had one white lady told me, say she sure wished I was workin' because she wadn't goin' to no hospital. 'Cause I've waited on her before. I don't know what she'll do. [They can *force* them to the hospital now.] And these clinics—now, some places, midwives can work in the clinic, but this one you can't. I had one lady came in—I could go to the clinic—I delivered a baby right there in the clinic because the lady didn't know she was gonna have the baby. [Laughter.] I delivered the baby, then I couldn't carry her to the hospital. [They just didn't know if they want ya.] That's wrong. If having your babies at home is your desire, [and] if you listen to these doctors, you'd be *afraid* to have it at home.

Ever deliver twins?

I delivered two sets of twins in one day.

What was that like?

Oooh! Beeeutiful! That was when I had my place out here. Was two little girls born out here, and before the day's out, there was a little boy and girl that was born down in W—— Park.

Same day?

Same day! I didn't get n'er bit of nothin'. [They woulda had a] write-up about it, look like, don't it? Two sets of twins in one day.

You must have had a hard time sleeping that night.

Oh, it's like when I go out to deliver a baby, when I come in, I just usually can't go to sleep. There's something about it that keeps you awake. But that day I was too tired. I couldn't do nothin' *but* go to sleep.

Tell me about an interesting birth you remember.

Well, I had one girl I delivered—now I've had all *kinds,* but she wouldn't stay in the bed. She wouldn't do nothin'; she just climbed and twist. I could never work with her; I went right along with her. She say, "Well, alright, I'm gonna go out the door." And I said, "Well, go ahead on; you'll come back." I didn't go out; I didn't follow her. She went out on the back porch; I stayed right there by that bed. And when the right pain hit her, she came back. [Laughter.] I've had 'em fightin', bitin', do everythin'.

What do you do with the women who fight against you?

I didn't do nothin' as long as I keep 'em in place right there where they had the baby. I didn't care what they do. I just wanted them to have the baby. The same stages gonna come; they ain't gonna do nothing but sit, go and lay down or sit down to where she can have the baby.

There's certain stages where they can't do anything but lay down?

That's right. But I had one lady, she never did lay down. She just stayed up and she walked, she walked. And I caught that baby—she was standin' up.

They say it's good for you to be able to walk around.

Oh, yeah, I let all mine walk.

Ever have a woman have one on her knees?

Oh, *lot* of 'em. It's hard hours—it's hard on you, but if you love the thing, then nothing's hard. But I've had a *lot* of 'em. Now, I had one lady who was gonna have a baby sittin'—had it on the waterbed. The last one I delivered, she was having it on the waterbed. I said, "Honey, wait a minute, you can't have no baby . . ." [Laughter.] So we got her out of bed; she fixed up a little [spot] on a rug on the floor, but it still wadn't hard enough for having a baby.

That is funny.

Yes, it is. On the waterbed? How do you . . .

You don't mind having fathers in the room?

I love having 'em. And I had one man, he said, "Well, I bet she won't have to have another baby." It looked like it be the worst thing he'd ever seen is her having a baby. [Laughter.] I said to myself, "We need more of you 'round here if that's gonna help."

Do you remember years ago when women had babies by midwife? You must have had your babies by midwife.

Yeah, I had a midwife. After my aunt died, in '50, and my baby was comin' in May, that's when she died, and I was so excited I was afraid to take it [with my baby]. But other than that . . .

All midwives?

Oh, yeah.

What's it like having a relative deliver your baby? Ever have your mother deliver you?

No. My aunt did.

It must be more comforting.

When they have their baby, I go there and get myself cleaned up and get them ready. If you can just sit down, and just rub 'em a bit, just do somethin', talk to 'em or pray—anything is a big help with having a baby. And I've never delivered very many babies that I wasn't sittin' on the side of the bed when the babies was born with my hand on their knee.

You massage them?

Oh, God, yeah, and put hot application, tell 'em to keep it there— that's good.

To keep from tearing?

If you can get some hot water, and just keep that water there, see, the skin expands.

It relaxes it?

It relaxes, mm-hmm.

And oil?

Yeah, massage 'em and oil 'em. And it's good. It allows you to examine them. You know what I mean? I would wash 'em up real good and get this oil and push it down there and just kinda get it to go down in there. Quite naturally, it would be easier for 'em. It's good. But they're theirs and not mine.

About the old days when a lot of women would be in the room— who was at your birth?

Let me tell you about one birth I had. When I went in there, they had sixteen people in the room. That was so. And then at least they had five men, and then they had *children* in there. And you know, they just got a lot of nerve; I couldn't do nothin'. I just couldn't do a thing. So one lady came on, and she cleaned the house out. And I was so glad, except one man, he wouldn't leave, and while she was having the baby, he stood up on the foot of the bed to get the pictures. That's another thing [I don't like]. But that was their business, see. But I didn't like that, he stood up and . . . No, somebody get the pictures; he [should've let her see the baby come]. But I've had several takin' pictures of the baby bein' born.

Some people are even doing video.

Yeah, I don't like that. I guess I'm old-fashioned. My pride. Lord, when all them peoples in that one little room.

How'd she do?

She didn't have no trouble. She *wanted* it to be, but I just didn't like that.

Too much confusion, too much noise?

Yeah, there's too much noise; there's too many people sittin' lookin' on. Now, I've lost cases by a lot of women. I've had *two* others that were carried right on to the hospital. They get the ladies excited. Well, you get them excited—ya know, talkin' and goin' on . . .

You can't concentrate.

No, God, I just don't want 'em standin' over me talkin' and goin' on; just let 'em go on. From then on, I did the lady's husband or friend—I did at least three would all be in there. 'Cause I'd say, "Get out." I delivered many babies by myself [with the mother]. I can do it myself. I know how to do it. It may take me a little longer like I've had no help to do nothin', but I don't know. I always could get around, see. The baby born; the mother had the baby; and then I wrapped the baby up and lay him aside, then I take care of the mother. If the baby's alright, then I keep an eye on him. I'd get the mother all straightened up, then I go and get that baby. Course I cut the cord after blood get to him. I wait so long; if I can do that, then I can be looking after her. That's another thing our mothers done good about goin' back to nursin' their babies. That's good. Oooh, I love to see 'em nurse their babies. You don't know what you gettin' when you buy this milk. One doctor to one of my patients, he told her he didn't want the baby to have that milk—that milk wasn't good for no baby. Yes, he did; I don't think that's right. I nursed *all* mine, every one of 'em.

Like we can improve on what's already there with a better product. You wonder what people have got in their heads sometimes.

Nothin'. [Laughter.]

Well, I hope one of your granddaughters takes it up.

I just hope so. Now mine—if I live long enough—mine may want to—the one in T—— now.

What school does she go to?

F——. All my children went to F——. All of them finished college, but the daughter, she came up in the day of the thirties. She didn't even finish high school. But she [learned] enough to go to New Jersey, and that's where she work now. Went to the hospital, and she got a lot of experience. She's been out there workin'. But I delivered a doctor's baby several years ago. She didn't want to go to the hospital. I waited on her.

Did you ever work with or know other midwives around town?

Yes, if I was at a place, someone had to take 'em. But I was so lucky. I had only two the whole time that I had to send to that I would be in some other place. But always, if I'm out, I'd leave the telephone number where I was gonna be so they could have help. This lady called—I was at [another birth]—and when she called, I was just about finished with that. I come on back out here on old W—— Road, and she had him within ten minutes after I got to the house. We stay in touch, you know.

Anyone name their baby after you?

Yes.

You keep track of any of those babies and know where they are or hear from them?

Yes. A lot of 'em's here in O——, and all over the world. But I meet so many grown men that say, "You delivered me." Some of 'em would be nice; some of 'em don't want nobody to know they used midwives. A lot of 'em don't want nobody to know. I had a little undertaker up here; he said he was born in O—— Memorial Hospital, and I *know* I delivered him. [Laughter.] They just don't wanta appreciate—they just think it's bad. It's what they are *taught:* a midwife is not wanted; she's not nothin'; you can't depend on 'em. But you can depend on 'em more than you can the doctor. My last baby was born here. That didn't give me a bad record. And because I wadn't expectin' her, I didn't have nothin' but newspaper. Normally, the pad, you know, you get from the house. But that's all they could see. And out there they takin' pictures.

Oh, and it didn't look good.

They had taken this when the people came to pick her up to take her to the hospital. That's when they take the pictures.

Why did they take pictures? They took pictures to hold against you?

Yeah. That's the only thing that I could see.

These were paramedics with the ambulance?

Yeah.

What year was that?

I guess that little baby about two years old.

This woman just showed up suddenly?

No, if I'd a known, if her mother'd been fair to me, if she hadda told me before that the placenta locked on her . . . Her placenta locked up—that's bad. She went home from the hospital and stayed ten days, and then she had to go back. But she went to the doctor. This doctor looked at her, but he didn't see no trouble. She didn't want to tell the truth. After that had happened, then she could have said, "I'm gonna take a chance." If she had told me, I wouldn't have gone into that. After that, we had to carry her on to the hospital.

So the whole reason you stopped your license . . .

That got on my nerves.

But nobody came to you and said you can't do it.

Oh, no, no, no. I've never had my license revoked in my life, and they've tried all kinds of ways to find something on me to keep me from workin'.

What else did they do?

I've had to come out on—you know, right on out—anything to come right on in. The nurses, they never was able to find anything. I had one little white girl, and her [placenta] locked on her; we sent her out to S—— Hospital. And when she went out there, they started bellyaching, and this doctor at the clinic, he stopped; he said that one doctor told him out there, he say, "It's not her fault." Said, "We just had one right here in the hospital, same thing." So he carried me of that, but they've been tryin' to get my license for a long time. I'd rather give it to them than to get it revoked. 'Cause I had a fifty-year license and never [had it revoked].

How long was your maternity home open?

About seven years.

What year did you close it?

I sure can't tell.

It's been within the last five, ten years.

Mm-hmm.

How many beds did you have?

I think I had five.

Did you have help?

Oh, yes. Now, I wouldn't have given it up, but you can't get no good help. People don't wanta work. On the weekends, I've had three or four people. And everybody would wanta come to work, but I'd do everything—give 'em a bath, feed 'em, change the bed, and cook.

What were you charging then?

Depended on what they get in for their check. I would get a check. I would get money out of their check—they didn't pay no extra.

You did all the washing, cooking; that was pretty much for free.

Well, it certainly were. Lot of work, but I like to work. Course with me now, soon as time you stop workin' . . . I've been tryin' somethin' to keep me together: some old person not treated very well, and I could just go and give 'em a lot of love, keep 'em alive. You need all the love you can get. Now, my daughter's up in New Jersey, her daughter don't treat her good at all. Just go off and leave her. She live in a house by herself. That's rough. She don't wanta come home. You know, she been sick so long up there with them doctors, she don't think she can live down here. I'm tellin' you. You just need love whether you're old or young. When you don't have no love . . .

I noticed how young and clear-minded the old, old midwives still are. I think that kind of work and their activeness has kept them that way.

Well, that helps a lot. If there's anything I enjoy, it's to see a baby come and to clean 'em up and dress 'em and get 'em ready and everything. And the mothers—I love to work with the mothers.

You just talk with them all night if you have to . . .

Sing, too. We'd just go through and go to sleep till they get in labor, 'cause lot of 'em's way off from home, and wait till the real thing comes along. Some of 'em call you before time. Stay there till the day and let 'em bring me home or stay till she get ready to have it. I still love it; I'll love it till I die.

I heard of this one blind midwife in Tennessee who people trusted more than the doctor about delivering babies. She just had the gift.

The gift. Now, if you got the gift . . . Mm-mmm, well, I'll tell you what, I delivered—I know you can't remember; it's before your time. You heard of the blackouts, when they wouldn't let you have lights in the house at night. I don't know if you heard about that. They was afraid to have lights in the house. And I delivered a baby during that without a light. I just felt my way. You got a guide; the Lord is with you, and you have a guide. You have somebody to teach you. I didn't get upset, but I've had mothers, you know, it would be gettin' on kinda rough at times. And I've had such a hard time, looked like we wasn't [prosperin'] and looked like the hours just . . . Ah, we'll take her to the hospital. And the Lord would put some light in my mind to do. I thank the Lord; every time I turn around, I'm thankful. He's been too good to me.

Don't you think that most of the midwives were church women?

Most of them. Though I have known one—a black girl—she wasn't no church woman. I tell you the truth. But *most* of us Christians. *Church* people—I don't know about the Christian.

So they were usually leaders in the church as well? Did other midwives talk to you about a calling, or did they just take it on?

Most of 'em just take it on that wants the job. A lot of people just like it. Just like now, there's a lot of people who would love to do that, but they won't give 'em a chance.

I wonder why people get it into their heads to do this—to change other people's work.

I know it, it's kind of a crooked world now. If one man can't get everything, he don't want the other man to have it. And that's bad. Just like the midwife. I could say something against one of 'em, but I never would because if I can't say something to help you, I wouldn't open my mouth. But after I helped this lady out, I'm gonna let a lot of 'em know that I'm gonna do trainin' because if we get [caught, they make us stop.]

Did you know of any midwives' licenses to be taken away unfairly?

No, I never known nobody. Not in this county. I've had a lot of complaints when they drink. Some of 'em'll drink. Oh, yeah. But I never drink.

A lot of them?

Not a lot, but once in a while you'll find one. There wasn't many. Now, I guess it's the same. I just never wanted to drink. Some of 'em drink. Just like doctors—you'd be surprised the way the doctors drink.

No, I wouldn't.

[Laughter.] That's right. Yes, sir, these doctors drink—some of 'em. A lot of 'em think it helps when they doin' somethin', but I didn't need that.

Maybe to get through a long labor. Did you have a period of con-finement that you would tell them to stay in bed for so many days?

No. My mother would make me stay in the bed nine days. When I got out, I was too weak to walk. And in them [days, they didn't let you] see no light; she was in a dark room. But now, these women now, there's one thing I object, but it doesn't do any good; they gonna do it if they want it: just as soon as the baby's born, they get up and get in the bathtub. I don't like it. It may not hurt; it's the way you were taught more than you feel about it.

So you don't think it makes any difference; they can get up when they feel like it?

Yeah, if they feel like it; if you strong enough, maybe get up, and I've known 'em to get up and go cleanin' the house. Some of 'em do that. I had one white girl out there had the baby, and her baby's three days old, and she was back out in the yard planting flowers. Now that was too early. I fussed at her, but it didn't do no good. [Laughter.]

Did you do a lot of work on the day of your births?

I worked. And I advise every woman who can do it to do it; it's good for her. My baby born the day I wake up.

It helps the birth come faster?

Yes, yes. See, some of 'em just lay around and do nothin', and that's harder. I was always active all my life. But I was workin' as a domestic servant when those white children were born. I was a midwife, but there wadn't no babies born in those times; times were hard. And I'd go to sleep and work and come home and have my baby.

Those were different times.

Oh, boy! Different people, too.

Do you think women were stronger then than they are now?

Mm-hmm, yeah. Because another thing I do now, if any mother have a baby, I put her on a band. I've had the nurses go right behind me and take 'em off of the mother and the baby, and I go right back and put 'em back on.

What are those for?

You know, you're all tumbled up in your stomach when you have a baby, and that holds you right together. Holds you and you can turn and do anything you wanted. The stomach just *hold* in. No, they don't believe in puttin' bands on 'em.

You never went to a midwife institute, just weekly meetings?

We used to have meetings once a month here, but the midwives would always meet up there. But we got to the place that we didn't want to go up there, and we didn't have nowhere to go, and this started happening before the midwives got away.

What kinds of things did they do at those meetings?

Just teach you what you were doin' and teach you what to do.

Were they generally right, or did you feel that some of the things they were teaching were—

Some of it was right; some of it . . . [Laughter]. You just pick up so much, ya know. 'Cause I always know mine. I wasn't ever no big ol' thing, but I always knowed my job.

I don't have any more questions. Can you think of anything we haven't talked about yet?

About they eatin'—that's another thing. They can eat, but you know . . .

Do you let them eat during labor?

Sure, if they feel like it. If you feel like it, you can eat all you want. But they won't let 'em eat; they say you don't need to eat. They wash the bowels out. You can do that if you want, but if they don't want it, don't do it. The fact about it is, they don't want all that to come [out on the bed]. But see, I make my own bedpan. And if they mess up, well, I can roll it up, put it out. Clean 'em up, and get on with it. If a lady has a baby and they won't let 'em eat after the baby's born, if the baby born tonight, you can't eat until tomorrow. Some of mine say, "I'm hungry." I say, "Well, alright. What do you want to eat?" I feed 'em. They *hungry;* they need to eat after the baby. They wouldn't let me have water. Mama wouldn't let me drink water. But that was *way* back then. Water don't hurt anybody. I don't believe in a whole lot of *ice* water.

Ice wouldn't hurt you, would it?

Too cold water might—probably would make you pain.

Cramp.

Oh, that's just old stuff, but I like it.

Was there a point in which there was a lot of pressure from other people for you to become a midwife?

Yeah, because they knew my people. The way I was acting, I guess they knew I would love it.

What do you mean they knew your people?

They knew my aunt was a midwife; she lived here, too, before she died.

And they figured if she was one—

Then *I* ought to be one. The doctors give me a good name on it for years and years. Even if a doctor don't like me, he'd always give me a good name; if he didn't like me, he didn't try to hurt me. When Dr. S—— came here, he tried to put [out] *all* midwives . . . He told us, said wadn't no midwives where he come from, and when he leave here, there wadn't gonna be none here. Now he told that. Honey, he been gone a long time, but I'm still here. I think it's ridiculous. That was real nasty. Now, I've had two white doctors was workin' with me but said they had to stop because if they work with *me*, they couldn't work in the hospital. Dr. B——, he worked with me, but Dr. C——, he just don't like the midwife. They was deliverin' their babies, but they had to stop—couldn't deliver they babies and do surgery, too.

I think a lot of this is also related to a scientific viewpoint.

Science has got things all messed up, too. A lot of things. That's another thing: with medicare, all of [you's got to pay for these] babies

to come in here. Well, that just keeps the midwives from [deliverin'].
One doctor say he think that if they pay the doctor, they should pay the
midwife; but they won't. We all deliver the baby. I just pray that we'll
all just pull together and try to help one another. Somebody gonna
have to; somebody gonna deliver, license or no license, one thing for
sure.

*Also, paramedics are allowed to deliver babies without any degree at
all. But they want the new midwives to have two years of nursing.*

One told me that he delivered six babies [that Monday] himself.
Now, see, that's unfair. He gonna deliver 'em, and he don't want us to
deliver. And we have our trade; [but I didn't go to] no school.

Do you think those monthly meetings were helpful at all?

I do believe they will, if we can get together. Only if we could get
some of the names of 'em, nearby. 'Cause we used to come as far as
T——, S——, all over the state once a month. If we could kinda get it
goin' for *someone* . . . Well, I don't know about if it's good or not to
have a license.

Do you think this bad treatment of midwives is rooted in racism?

Well, then, I don't say, it might be. But from the beginnin', they
probably get better trainin' 'cause if they go to school, some of 'em
don't take the time they *should* take. It's kind of a mixed-up thing. But
money is the beginning of all of it—everything else you can mention.
All the countries you ever come from—why not give a black one a
chance? We've done some good work. But they practice—you know
what I mean, they're bein' taught. So let's give everybody a chance.

A lot of midwives seemed to like those monthly meetings.

Yeah, it had to talk about different things. It's helpful to you, a help to *you*. They can tell me somethin' I know that I don't. That would be good if we could sort of get it goin'. *Most* people that have a baby, they don't want to be bothered with the fella that doesn't have anything, you see. That's bad. We just need to get a little closer together. I know two or three of these young womens would love to come on. They might have to go to school to do it. I thank God that I didn't have to. But you know, a nurse told me—now, I know she was wrong—other foreign countries mostly have cut out the midwife, but I don't believe her. I wish I could go work in a clinic. I wouldn't want a whole lot of mothers. Give me a little somethin' so that I can be there to enjoy the work. Now, Rebecca, she was so nice to me; she has sent here so many patients. She's a nurse-midwife.

And she was sending you some patients?

She *did* send. She was a very sweet midwife.

A young woman?

No, she's a foreigner. Oh, she had a lot of patients. But she went up—one lady went up to fourteen hundred dollars. And that don't hit the doctor's [fee], but it's much more than she was chargin' when she was workin'. She had to get out of O—— County. Start being a mess, you got to be gettin' permission from a doctor to deliver a baby. That was a mess, too. If he don't say you can, you can't. Something aggravate the devil out of ya. And then you got to call today so they can go in and investigate. That's the way they had it. I'll be so glad when one was born on a Friday, then I couldn't call it in till Monday. Everybody got to be real nasty. Well, we got a lot to learn and a lot to do, but they don't wanta do it. Now, what's wrong with me going in and birthin' babies? I don't know. And the ladies say they feel so good when they have it. It's not like being in that hospital—all them people; this one comin' to see about you, this one comin' and leavin'. They didn't take my license, now, but I just give it up because I just got tired of it. I don't care from now on. They have been trying to catch me deliverin' babies since I retire. I know they doin' it. I had one one night call me, said, "Well, I came out there to see you." I say, "I'm sorry, but I sure can't wait on you." That was a catch. There was something about it, the Lord [made me see] it was happenin'. I had another come in here wantin' to know if I could wait on her. You know, she got all the information she could, and I haven't seen her since. So I didn't do the job; it came to *me* before the baby's born not to go. Somethin' against ya. They got to have proof. You have to watch 'em. And I wouldn't try to harm 'em; I would not harm anybody. We got some terrible people around here.

I guess you never imagined when you started midwifing that you'd someday be an outlaw, did you?

Oooh! Idn't that the truth! I just worked for the county, I used to work for the city. People didn't have money in the county. Eight or ten dollars—till the money came in 'cause there wadn't no money in it then. 'Cause they didn't have all these things they have at the hospital now. Them doctors is workin' for money; the midwife didn't.

Did they try to get you all to wear masks?

Oh, yeah . . .

You didn't do that, did you?

No. [Laughter.]

[Looking at a newspaper article about her practice.] This is funny what you said: "I think it's better for the fathers can be there all

they want, and they usually try to help, but they aren't worth too much, to tell you the truth." You delivered your own baby one night.

I delivered three of mine.

Oh, when you said that earlier, I thought you meant you delivered three of your kids' babies.

My husband's cousin; she was there to assist me if I needed anything.

You did it on your knees?

No, in the bed.

Interview with Rosalind Stephenson, March 1983

> Mrs. Stephenson is a seventy-one-year-old black midwife from rural north Florida. She has been midwifing for thirty-four years and has a set of triplets to her credit.

But the doctors say they ain't gonna have nothing to do with us—the midwives.

Because of the new law?

The new law. My baby girl, my last one, she born in '49. I been a midwife ever since then, and I ain't never had no trouble. And if it wadn't for just they can, say, sue ya, whether it's somethin' *I* did or somethin' just happened to the patient, I wouldn't even count it.

'Cause somebody out there need us midwives. Hell, everyone not able to go to the hospital. Us ain't catchin' no babies no how since the welfare took over. We don't catch no babies.

When was your last delivery?

In January this year. Now, you know that ain't catchin' no babies. Most of them go to the hospital, and the girls will tell ya, "Miss Rosalind, we don't need you no more. I'm on welfare, and the welfare pay for my baby." Mm-hmm. See, they won't bill us midwives if us waitin' on one.

When did that start?

Oh! Ever since I've been on. Ever since they started welfare. So these people don't pay for no babies. Only way we get a chance to wait on anyone is just like if a grandmother gonna pay for her daughter if she got pregnant. Now, that's the po' grandmother got to pay, and she haven't been on welfare. But just as quick as that baby born, then she [the mother] go get on welfare; then they go to takin' care of her. And she just continue to get babies and babies and babies 'cause the welfare gonna pay for it. You know, the checks for the babies and all that. So if I had to just, say, live on what I catch babies, I'd have been dead. I said I want you to come and talk with me, but I ain't gonna put myself up in that. Elizabeth and me is the only ones; Johnnie and Roberta, they is still for it. But I'm not.

I know of two women from the next county going over to Johnnie's house for deliveries.

Nuh-uh, Johnnie don't supposed to be deliverin' at her house, 'cause I used to deliver here, and they say you got to have *two* bathrooms.

And I said, "Well, I ain't got no two bathrooms." That's what the health department lady said. "Rosalind, you must have two bathrooms." Elizabeth went and had her another bath put in. I said, "Well, I'm not able to do that."

When did she tell you that?

Oh, last year when us went there finding out about, you know, could us deliver at home. I even had a big room back there for my folks. I had it built for that. And she told me, she said, "Rosalind, you can't have no more deliveries at your house"—Miss M—— and the lady what was from Jacksonville.

Wonder where that rule came from?

I don't know. 'Cause I feel that I could do what I want under my house. 'Cause if they get sick, I did have some girls here deliver. Let me see, what was it? I couldn't get the afterbirth, the placenta. And I carried 'em to the hospital. So the doctor done it. Things done changed so much till I'm not . . .

I need to talk to Miss M—— at the health department to find out what the rules are.

She say she don't know nothing there. What upset her so, they was sending us all these papers. And Miss M—— said, "Well, y'all got me behind." When the lady come from Jacksonville, we thought it time for her to come and be with us. So she come, and Miss M—— said, "Now, all these midwives comin' in throwin' this in *my* face, and I don't know nothin' about this law." And say, "I figured y'all should have brought it to me—sent *me* a paper." And so Miss M—— didn't like it a bit. I think this was the last one they sent us. It was; that's the last one; this was the first 'un. [She hands me a technically worded, mimeographed, multipaged copy of new HRS rulings on midwifery in Florida.] And Miss M—— was mad about it. Say, "Now, I don't know nothin' about all this, Miss R——." When the lady come, us had to carry 'em all back over there. She said, "The laws in these papers, is that what you mean for us to go by? And if us thinks us can't do it, us got to give up us license and give up our papers." 'Cause all that junk what is tellin' about what you got to do, and Miss M—— say, "Uh-uh, I'm not gonna let my midwives go through with nothin' like that."

There are no new midwives coming up, are there?

Oh, no, no. They ain't takin' on no midwives. They ain't but us.

There are some young midwives in T—— that want to start practicing. They are having a hard time. They changed these rules thinking it would help them, but now they're not so sure.

You know, a bunch of 'em wanta come, and when I have a delivery, want me to carry 'em out with me. They say they have to go out with ya about five times, or something like that. And then for her to approve that she was with her, and she have to kind of demonstrate some things what I did when I was deliverin'. So they said, no, that wouldn't be. If they want to be a midwife, now they have to go to the hospital and take training. Yes, all the ladies go down there to T—— to the health department. It was a lady in Georgia. She was out in the field like we was. But she said, "Mis' Stephenson, they cut all us midwives off from out here in L—— County. Only way now I can deliver—I have to be here to the hospital to deliver." We've known a lot in Georgia.

Do you understand what happened? It seems pretty tricky.

Ain't it, though? When they got up all this tricky mess, I wanta trick right out. 'Cause you don't have no secret if your group is perfect when you have it inspected. And the doctor, when they turn 'em loose from the health department and say are we in a position to wait on 'em, that been all to it. But now you got to go through us doctor, sit down with us patient, find out do you got high blood [pressure], is anybody in your family ever had TB, has anybody in your family ever had syphilis. You know they's not gonna tell you. They're not gonna tell you. When they go to the health department and be examined when they start bein' pregnant, it they place to find out all that. 'Cause we can't wait on 'em, not a one, till they turn 'em loose from the health department or either from the doctor.

You don't have to go for your annual physical any more?

Mis' M—— told us, say, "No, us don't have to come there no more for havin' things like that." But we have to go to the doctor's if us want a physical. She has no more to do with us.

Did she lose her job?

Miss M——'s still around, but she's not in possession of us. Just like if you was over the midwives, we'd go in there and get information from you for you to tell us what must be did and everything. But they ain't givin' Miss M—— that privilege no more. If we wait on one, we fill out our own birth certificate blank and carry it into the health department. That's all they got to do. They'll still take the birth certificates when us carry 'em in, but that's all the health department's got to do with us. Talk to them and find out, and then you can explain it to the midwives out here. You will know more about gettin' it from them, 'cause Mis' M—— told us like this: She said, "It's up to y'all; you're on your own." She said, "I'm mighty afraid some of y'all's gonna be messed up.

You're gonna be sued for nothin'. Somebody's gonna tell a lie and say, 'Aunt Rosalind delivered my baby, and I caught some germs or somethin'.' " But, see, they don't go into these homes. Sometimes I carry my own sheets and things, somethin' clean to lay on. A lot of us midwives do. 'Cause if we was to lay our babies on what they have in they homes sometimes, we *know* the baby's gonna get it. I have even went to the white folks and told them, said—so many roaches all in the bed, waterbugs—I said, "The baby's gonna die unlessen you send somebody there to spray that house." And the man sent sombody there and say, "Mis' Stephenson, tell 'em is there anywhere they can go and stay until we spray the house." I say, "I'll carry 'em somewhere." So I carried them to the daughter's, and they sprayed the house. See, but they put it all on the *midwives*. Things [at] home have to be sufficient sometime for you to deliver a baby.

So everything was fine. You were practicing until last January about a year ago?

Yeah. Everything's *still* fine, but Miss M—— ain't told us nothin'. They had a midwife meetin' last Tuesday. I was on my way goin' to the meetin', and a deer hit my car, and I couldn't go, and I called there and told her. So she said, "Well, Mis' Stephenson, I'm glad you didn't get hurt, but I kinda enlighten ya on some of the things what they had in the meetin' if they have it." That was what Mis M—— say.

How did you learn to be a midwife?

I was goin' around practicin' to be a midwife before '49. And Mis' Ellen Harmon supposed to be carryin' me around with her until I could go around with her five times. And so she wouldn't never call nobody. If the peoples was pregnant, and I found out Mis' Ellen was goin' to wait on 'em, I'd sneak in, 'cause see, she's scared if they get another midwife; it would cut her out some of the people. And so my cousin Vanessa, she was pregnant, and she told me, said, "Rosalind, I'm gonna let you deliver my baby." I said, "I ain't got my equipment yet." She says, "That's alright. Let me run this risk." And she let me. She said, "Go up there and get you my number-eight spool of thread." And I got the number-eight spool of thread. She said, "Double it." It was about that long. I tie a knot in the end, put the two ends together, and chunk 'em in the pot. I tied three of 'em and throwed 'em in the pot. She said, "Now put the scissors in the pot and boil it. And when the baby comes, then you just take somethin' and take 'em up. Don't put your hand on 'em, and let you cut it." So when the baby born, she let me wait it on her with her daughter.

Were you by yourself?

I was by myself. 'Cause when I got through, she told her husband to go get Mis' Eliza Overton—'cause she was the *old* midwife—to come and see that I fixed up everything alright. So Mis' Eliza come, and she seen how I had did and dressed the baby's navel and all.

That's what the thread was for?

Yeah, to tie the cord. So Mis' Eliza said, "What'd you send for me? She did it just as good as I'd a did it." I tried to get Mis' Ellen to show me how to fix up the birth certificate. So she wouldn't show me. Miss W——, she fixed it up for me. I had wrote it on a piece of paper, everything what the mother told me—the baby's name and everything, what time the baby born. Then Miss W—— fixed it up. Dr. W—— signed it; he sent it on for me and say, "Go over to the health department and tell 'em *I say,* 'I built this clinic in H—— and let you be—give you your license.' " So that's how I got my license.

Why wouldn't the midwife fill it out for you?

She didn't want me to be a midwife. She was an old lady, and she think that I was goin' to take some of her patients. And so ever since then, when they start to meetin', I been goin' to the meetin' and learnin' more and more about it.

There's always something new to learn?

No, they just told us how to make beds, how to prepare a bed when you get ready to deliver, and how to, you know, shave the lady when you get ready.

You have to shave them now?

Yes. Just 'round the birth canal. [This midwife later told me that she didn't think shaving the woman was necessary and tells her mothers to just tell the health department at the postnatal examination that the baby came so fast they didn't have time to shave her.]

Do you have any relatives who are midwives?

My grandmother was a midwife, my auntie was a midwife, and I wanted to be a midwife.

Because of them?

Oh, yeah. You know, when I was growin' up, I always said that I wanted to be a midwife. So I got to be it. The next thing I said, "Lord, now you done blessed me to be a midwife. I got *that* job." I said, "Now, the next thing I want in life is to go around and see after old people and show the people how old folks should be treated." So now I got that! I work five hours goin' around cleanin' up old folks' houses and fixin' their breakfast. If they need bathin', I'll bathe 'em. And so I just can't do nothin'.

If someone came to you now and wanted you to deliver their baby, you would have to say no?

I can't serve 'em if I don't have my license. See, us licenses out in December, the thirtieth.

You're not going to renew?

I don't know. I fill out my blank and send it off. Now, I don't know if they gonna still give them any license. Some of 'em says us got to pay for 'em. But from what I saw on the paper, if that's all us got to pay for 'em—five dollars—I don't care. I don't mind payin' it, but, you know, if you don't catch no more than one baby a year, they figure you don't need no license. That's why I say I didn't have but two babies to turn in. One for '81 and one for '82. So I don't know as I'm gonna get any.

They have those midwife meetings just once a month?

Us have 'em once a month. The last day in every month. If it on a Saturday, us have it that Friday. She [the county nurse] just sit around and tell us things, then show us pictures of different things, you know, what has to be done. They show you all that in a picture. And we know if the blood high, it teaches us you can't wait on 'em. When we shave 'em down there, if we see any kind of little sore or anythin', you know not to wait on 'em.

So you think the meetings were good?

Yes! Us loves our meetings.

Who delivered your baby for you?

Mis' Ellen. Mis' Ellen had us deliver my baby.

Did she deliver all your babies?

She delivered my second child and my last one. They wasn't takin' nobody to no hospitals.

There was no hospital in your county?

I never had no nothin'. Yeah, there might have been, but we didn't— uh-uh. These people go to the hospital now is just because they don't have to pay! Reagan cut out that welfare and all this different things. *He* doesn't wanta have the babies at home. Now, I had two white ladies from T—— to call me, askin' me will I deliver their babies. But I told 'em I can't come in there. That's what gets me when you say Johnnie takin' some. I could've got them, but the lady told me, said, no, she had three children and she'd prefer to have her babies at home.

The one she had was a long time ago; it was over a year. And this other one hasn't had hers yet. She may not make it out there.

Well, she ain't gonna do it. Johnnie done know better. She know she can't get nobody from T——. Now they come to some of they *people's* house in G—— County here, we can wait on 'em.

The woman is going through the G—— County Health Department.

Well, that's right. That's why she can wait on 'em. She can wait on 'em. If she was goin' over there to a doctor in T—— or to the clinic over there, then she couldn't. She could wait on 'em if she was goin' over there to the health department.

What would you require to be a midwife if it were up to you?

Well, I don't think they're supposed to be goin' out no five times. No, I don't. No, that's too many. If the [experienced] midwife was to sit down and talk to the new midwife and have her with her on about three cases, I feel like she ought to be willin' to can do that. 'Cause you know, the biggest thing it is, is learnin' 'em how to massage that stomach, harm [*sic*] that placenta outta the baby. You got to really know how. Some of [the mothers will] shove your hands back, but you can't let 'em do it. You got to keep on rollin' and rubbin' until that thing get hard as 'dis [knocks on wooden table]. And after it get hard, you ain't got nothin' to fear. 'Cause some of 'em, by the time somebody holler at 'em, "Don't hurt my stomach!" they quit. But you can't do it. You're gonna have to keep on 'cause you the one doin' the workin'; you've got to carry things out right.

What do you think about all these women wanting to go back to midwives now?

That's right, that's right. And I'm glad. I'm glad!

But some doctors want to keep this from happening.

Yes, there is. That's what I told 'em. All of them, but we can fight this thing 'cause, child, you know, *everybody* ain't able to go to that hospital. Like I hear them say they done gone up on [the cost] for bein' in the hospital for one day. Ain't nobody can pay no hundred dollars a day for bein' in the hospital. So that's why I say, these women, they have their babies, they keep 'em there, don't know how long. Some of 'em was on welfare, they let 'em go through in three days. Well, there's somebody what ain't on welfare, they keep 'em there a long time. Why they can't let *them* go home and keep down a bill? But see, they know that somebody got money, mm-hmm. But you *need* your money. If you let her went home in three days, why can't I go home in three days? If the people was lookin' to it and *fight* this thing, and just if so many people decide that they still want the midwives on, we can fight it.

When you were a girl, and there were a lot more midwives, did people look up to the midwives in those days? What kind of women were they? Church women?

That's right. They was church women. They had a lot of confidence in 'em. I don't have to tell it, but since you want me to explain, you could ask white, black, any of 'em. Ask 'em, say, "If you was to have a midwife, who would you rather have just right 'round in H——?" They'll say, "Send me Rosalind." Mr. Spence Booth, when he had his farm goin', he tell 'em, say, "Now, if you gonna have that baby, you better speak to Rosalind. 'Cause Rosalind say you got to go to the hospital, I'm gonna send you. But if she say you can have your baby, I ain't sendin' you to no hospital." And I'm tellin' you, he'd tell any of 'em, say, "Rosalind's a good 'un." Yeah, 'cause Joannie, the girl over there named Joannie Hanson, I think she's got seven or eight children, and I waited on her with every one of 'em 'cept one. [Laughter.]

Do the children grow up knowing you're the one who delivered them?

Uh-huh. Oh, I got a bunch of children around here.

Do people ever call you for any other kind of health problems?

Yes, they call me. A lady called me the other week here, say, "Mis' Rosalind, they say you good on rubbin' folks and puttin' their body up. Could you help me?" I say, "Yes, but I'm not allowed to do that no more." I say, "They don't allow us to do that no more. But you just lay flat on your back. Let your head hang down, lay in the chair, and let somebody get in and just take your stomach just like this. Just reach down in there and pull and come over like you're gonna fold this thing 'round your navel, and then let somebody rub your stomach with a little Vaseline and powdered [alum] and band yourself up." So she [did that], but don't tell nobody! [Laughter.] So she talk like this, she say, "Oooh, Mis' Stephenson, uhh! That mornin' I got up I didn't feel like anything." They don't allow us to do that no more. Yeah, I had 'em laughin' the other day, I say, "Lord, when that bump dance come out, I had me a heap o' people to wait on 'cause them girls'd go out and bump 'em with them high-heeled shoes on. [And one night I'd] doctor 'em for their stomach." [Laughter.]

Some women have talked of midwifery as a calling. What do you think of that?

Well, I don't know about all that, but I do know if anybody got a strong belief in you and feel like you gonna try to do somethin' to help 'em, they'll call on you regular. That's the way I feel about it. But this here God callin' and all that, it's just somethin' you want to *do,* and if you wanta do a thing, when you do it, you wanta do it right.

Did your grandmother being a midwife have something to do with you wanting to be one?

I don't know, but I just been wanta be one. I just felt like there's *somebody* got to do somethin'. I'm gonna die one day, and I can be a help to somebody. And so out of my auntie dying, my grandma dying . . . This what worry me now: they cut out all the midwives, who is goin' to help these poor peoples what not able? That's the way I feel about it. *Somebody* got to do somethin'. If they ain't got no money, and they done cut out all the midwives, that's more money the government got to pay out. I ask the lady what come out, I say, "What do the doctors charge to deliver a baby?" She say, "Twelve hundred dollars." I say, "Now, that's them! That's what they say they charge." I say, "But down here they got to set our price for we to go out and deliver a baby—a hundred twenty-five dollars. Now, ain't that somethin'?" I say, "You oughta see yourself; they don't want us midwives. The reason they don't want to help us out, they want everything comin' they way; the more midwives is cut out, them what us been waitin' on, *they* can get 'em." That's twelve hundred dollars, when we can go out there and help somebody for one little ol' hundred twenty-five dollars. Sometime we don't [even] get that. We just went out there and wait on 'em. But the reason they don't call on me, 'cause I tell 'em, "You better not call me. When you call me and engage me, be sure you be bringin' my money and start puttin' it down." I got a book in there when they's payin' twenty-five dollars. I got so many peoples owe me. But when they went up to forty dollars, don't nobody owe me. When they went up to fifty dollars, don't nobody owe me. Look like when they went up, they paid better. 'Cause I got on that scale like Mis' M—— told us, said, "Do like the doctor, let 'em start payin' on the deal when they engage ya." So I did.

You have some books from when you were a midwife a long time ago? You have a manual?

Oh, yeah! Mine done tore all the back off and some of the leaves out of it. Ain't nothin' changed but this new law right there. They tellin' you what you must do, go and sit down; I don't know if that's the paper, but she supposed to bring us a paper. They carry it and read it to 'em when they engage us if they had any kind of them diseases or anything. But it may not be in this one, but this the law here. 'Cause Mis' M—— say she didn't know nothin' about this. "Mis' Stephenson," she say, "I'm sorry. You're the second one done brought all this paper in here to me. It was mailed to you from Jacksonville." The other lady [from the state office] typed 'em and fixed 'em up, and since [then] they sought a date for her to come out and explain [the new law] to her [Miss M——]. Mis' M—— said, "I would like to sit in, too, and listen." So after she got through talkin', Mis' M—— say, "Well, you ain't got me nowhere in the record—in the plan. Who gonna be over my midwives?" She said, "Nobody!" Said, "They don't need you over them." She still work there, but she ain't got nothin' else to do. Mis' M—— say, "They not goin' to have the meetings like they been havin' once a month?" She say, "No." "Bag inspection?" "No!" I can't tell you nothin' but just how I started to be a midwife and how I'm *so rarin'* to continue to be a midwife, but we got to go by these laws. And if us got to go by them laws, we *need* a doctor or someone to back us up or be behind us. And if I deliver a baby and the baby is not normal, I suppose to rush and carry it to the health department, then they takes over. But no more. They ain't got no more to do with us. Us on us own. So I didn't go to the last meeting. But I really hope you will talk with her [Miss M——] and then come back a day if you can next week and say, "Well, Mis' Stephenson, I did go." 'Cause I don't want to get off. But this thing about you're on your own; if anything come up, no doctor's gonna help you; they can sue you. I'm on and they're off. [Laughter.] 'Cause my husband gone, and I worked too hard for my home, and I ain't gonna let nobody take it. [At this point, I called Miss M—— from Mrs. Stephenson's home.]

Miss M—— doesn't sound like she plans to give up. She said you would get your license right on in January.

She say she gonna fight like the devil 'cause she feel like they should have somebody over us.

How old is she?

She's a young lady. She's from [a Northern city]. She's the onliest one older that could get in Miss H——'s place. She's the only one's had, you know—I forget what you call it . . .

Seniority?

Yeah. To take over. So after they offered her that much money, that's why she don't be wantin' nobody but herself; she said she don't want no one comin' and her losin' her job 'cause G—— County payin' her nicely. But it wadn't doin' nothin' 'bout she wantin' to talk with her midwives and things. 'Cause we had been all raisin' cancer money. She'd lighten us up on that, but some of 'em still do it. We midwives raised a thousand dollars on the cancer drive. They give the party over there to the bank. They wasn't gonna invite us 'cause us was black faces. They give us a brass pin and an ink pen. She said, "Girls, I'm tellin' ya, I don't wanta come here and stop y'all, but y'all just reachin' at them people." Say, "Each one has so much they turn in every year, and y'all just went overboard. Then they didn't think enough to invite y'all."

Is she black?

She black. "Didn't even think enough to invite y'all in." And I just cut off 'cause I figured if I done run 'round here and *begged* and helped raise money, they could've let us come in and been in with the party.

Do you have any papers from your grandmother's time of her practice?

No, I don't. I just wisht I could've got some of my auntie's papers. She had a doctor book and everything. And I wanted the book so bad, but my cousin—I don't know who she done with it. After she died, the old man was stayin' with her just got rid of everything. They just started that junk about cuttin' out midwives. They just started that. But still whatever we got to do, we're gonna do it. That's how come I tell ya it ain't all that hard. Onliest thing what botherin' me, we've got to have a doctor say, "Well, when things get so y'all can't handle 'em with a patient, then bring 'em in to us." That's all I want 'em to say. That's all. 'Cause there is some time when you're deliverin' a baby, somethin' come up and you need somebody a little higher than you. So if they just agree to do that, they couldn't *stop* me. I *love* it. Everybody say, "Rosalind, you love to midwife?" I *love* it. It's doin' somethin' to help somebody. I done did it so much it don't worry me none. I done waited on my cousin, and her baby was deformed. Now, I had to go through some real hard [deliveries], but I didn't mind. 'Cause, see, when a baby come not right, we have to report it to our health department. The baby's skin was just like hardened. When I lay it down, the foots go way back behind the head, and if I sit 'em up, they . . . [She drops her hands.] I don't know whether the child was just messed up. So I just turn in that somethin' was wrong. And they told me to tell the mother to bring it to the health department.

Did it live?

Yes. Still livin'! Caroline's little girl.

What's your bedside manner like, what kinds of things do you do?

I just sit and wait. Sometimes they often have a pain. You know, I may catch the knees and kinda press against her like that, but it's nothin' there if you don't rub 'em. 'Cause you may rub 'em, and the baby get [crossways]. So you not allowed to rub. If anything, just press and tell her how to pant.

You let them walk around?

I don't want 'em to get in the bed, but some of 'em *want* to get in the bed. Then when that time come, they *have* to be in the bed, they wanta get up. I say, "I told ya to stay up—long as you walk, just stay up and walk." But now, "Mis' Rosalind, I got to lay down!" When that time comes, I don't have no trouble with 'em 'cause they say, "Oh, God, don't get that woman. That woman gonna *make* you get back in that bed." Oh, yes.

Have you had any have their babies on their knees?

Yes, I have, but that is so dangerous for 'em to do it, to get on their knees to have the baby.

Why?

I don't know, but see, if they laying down, I just had to cut it out. I used to say, "I'll let you work in your own convenience." But you can't *do* that. 'Cause if I let 'em work to their own convenience, some of 'em say, "Well, can't I turn on my side?" I say, "Now, ain't that stupid!" [Laughter.] I just goes on and tell 'em. Oooh, me and my girls have it! When they get mad at me, "Rosalind, I'm sorry if I made ya mad and everythin'." [Laughter.]

Have you got an unusual story you want to tell me?

One girl, me and her grandmother was waitin' on her, and the girl went in her room and locked the door. [Laughter.] When she locked the door, she had a pain. "Ah! Mis' Rosalind, come 'ere, come 'ere." I say,

"Uh-uh! You done locked me out. I ain't comin', I ain't comin'." "Mis' Rosalind, won't you get in my room!" I say, "I ain't comin' *nowhere!*" Ooooooh! When that pain was up, I bet she didn't lock that door no more. [Laughter.] Oh, I have so much fun with 'em.

What about having fathers in the room at the birth?

They like it, but I don't. See, I just don't be wantin' 'em in there. But they showed a picture to us over there, say it helps the mother, and then I believe it do 'cause one girl was over there on the other side of Q——, and I waited on her. She was single, and it was her boyfriend. She said, "Mis' Rosalind, let my boyfriend come in. He can help me, and I'll have this baby." I said, "Oh, you gonna have this if the boyfriend don't come in. Go on and have that baby!" That boy come in there and on his knees and throwin' his hands up under that girl's back, and God knows, the baby come *so* quick. I say, "Now, you is going to make me believe in this here." She said, "Well, I *told* you he could help me."

Why don't you like fathers in there?

I just be 'shamed in there. I just be 'shamed that they be in there. 'Cause, see—have you seen a baby born? This way I be thinkin' the boy gonna be teasin' her. I don't be wantin' 'em to see nothin' to tease their girlfriends or their wives. We never know these men! They're liable to get [hard and come up here any times and make us hurt 'em.] Make their *wives* hurt 'em. 'Cause if [they] have a little fallin' out, he may tease that girl or his wife. And that's why I don't like 'em or want 'em in there.

Do you let their mothers come?

Oh, yeah! The mother, the sister, [or] if they got a little friend lady. But the rest, they say, "Oh, Mis' Rosalind ain't gonna let nobody in the room with ya." So I say, "Now if you got a friend, she can come in and help ya." But all this other crew runnin' in to see a baby born, they gettin' out. Wait till they have theirs, and then they'll see it. I don't care. They know me—I won't play it.

Did you want to add anything we haven't said yet?

Ain't nothin' *I* wanta say, but just say this: How in the world do y'all expect for the midwives to work for you if you ain't givin' 'em no backup nowhere? Say they don't know if they gonna have any problems. So if they have a problem, why don't some of ya tell us or tell them that you are willing to help 'em out. That's all I be want 'em to do. And everything will roll on. They should *know this. You* know it! Many young girls havin' babies now, [and] everybody not able to go to that hospital. 'Cause the man sure gonna cut 'em all off. He cuttin' 'em like mad offa that welfare, and somebody got to help these children. The midwives—here us old, us know, but now they talkin' about them what trainin', I'm sorry for 'em. 'Cause if they gonna go to the hospital and be trained, no midwife's gonna hardly help 'em.

You think it's better to be trained by a midwife?

To the hospital. See, this is what we say. They had 'em over here to the health department. I'll tell you just like I told them: why am I gonna train you, and I'm already knowin' you turnin' me off? I ain't gonna help train you nothin'. That's the way *I* am. They get over there—wanta go out with us on a case. 'Cause I ain't carryin' [them] out with me. They tellin' me they gonna turn us off. And these girls us training are gonna take us place. Let the hospitals train 'em. Let 'em be trained to the hospital.

Did you ever go to any of those midwife institutes at FAMU?

No, no, no. I know they had some over there.

What did you hear about them?

Esther Barton, she went to 'em when she was gettin' on to be a midwife. And who else it was? Martha, but Martha off now. She's a young girl; they turned her off. They went over there. This is what you talkin' about—trainin' to get 'em to be a midwife. Esther Barton went 'cause she didn't have no midwife around her to take her out, and somebody else they sent to Sanford. I don't know who that was—a lady down there to a maternity home. They sent 'em down there to stay, I think it was a week, and took training.

Did they say they were good?

Oh, yeah, it was good.

                    *   *   *   *   *

[A story about triplets]

The girl didn't have no hot water. The mother went over there and come back with a pan of hot water. So when she come, I say, "Now, Pam, this stupid gal got *two* babies!" She had the pan of water. "What you say, Rosalind?" I say, "She got twins!" [Claps her hands.] Just dropped the whole pan of water. [Laughter.] And I was so tickled, you know? "Bless your soul." I say, "You get out from here and go get me some more water." [Laughter.] She went and get some more water. When she come back, I said, "*Pam!* Here *another* baby!" "Oh, god-damn!" [She acts out dropping the pan again.] Mr. Spence Booth and them—they had the pictures took.

Is that who it was, Mr. Spence's daughter?

No, no, the girl stay on his place. She was named Marty Kenny. And honey, that woman, her momma tickled me so bad. [Laughter.] I can't help it—a crazy lady—just dropped *all* the water. I say, "You better go ahead just get those sheets and wrap my babies up." And they looked so pretty. So *I* wanted to have on my cap and my apron and be there *with* the babies, but they went and had the babies' picture made and put it in the papers.

Appendix

A Long Dark Night

The Midwives of Florida

by David K. Fulton

David Fulton, a Florida public health worker, wrote "A Long Dark Night" around 1920 as a proposal for a book on midwives in Florida that was never completed. As he notes elsewhere, "each chapter will consist of two parts, the first dealing with the fictional Mattie and her friends, the second being the factual history of that period of time in Florida midwifery." Unfortunately, Fulton's writing fails to provide "factual history" in either the first or second chapters. He presents no statistical foundation for his assertions and makes sweeping generalizations.

A tiny yellow flame danced wearily among the red embers in the fireplace. The room was filled with an age-old darkness that the people in it did not sense, for they were a part of it. The three other women who were on their knees praying, while Mattie leaned close over the still figure on the bed. "Lawd, he'p me—he'p me," she mumbled fervently over and over. The screams had stopped and the writhing of the child—for that was all she was—had ceased. Mattie put her face down against the black nose, and felt of the sweat-soaked chest for signs of life. The little yellow flame danced no more. The embers were a deep red like the last faint glow of a sunset.

Mattie straightened slowly and looked at the others. There were no words. She bent again and covered the girl with a dirty sheet. The tragic mound made by the unborn child in her abdomen showed starkly. Mattie looked again at the others. Her shoulders slumped. Her stocky ebony body quivered with the exhaustion of her fruitless vigil. She picked up a rag and began to wipe the blood from her hands. From the corner came the ancient wail of her people, as the two older women, mother and grandmother, swayed forward and back—forward and back—palms raised, chanting the wordless mourning for the dead.

The third woman sat and stared across the room. Twenty or so, for nobody knew, tall and spare like her father, she ignored her sister on the bed, her Aunt Mattie, her mother and grandmother, and seemed to be unaware of her surroundings. Her head was lifted slightly, and her intelligent face showed no emotion, but it was the only live thing in the room that Mattie could turn to in her plight. "Mary Jo," Mattie said, "get yo' fathah."

Mary Jo rose without a word, and walked slowly toward the door of the one-room cabin. She stopped as both women heard the man's heavy step on the porch. Then they both stepped forward quickly to meet him outside. Mattie shivered as the cold early-morning air bit through her sweat-soaked clothes.

Joe Parker, perhaps forty-five, was a big man and powerful. His six-foot-four frame was draped with the muscles that bespoke his years of hard labor, and the jet-black skin that told of his Sudanese ancestry glowed in the faint glimmerings of the dawn. He looked at his daughter and sister-in-law.

"Ah huhd de mo'nin'," he rumbled, and his face clouded. "Ah'm gonna fin' dat boy—"

"No use talkin' lak dat, Joe," Mattie said softly. "Young'uns is dat way. Dis gonna happen sometimes."

Joe was not a violent man. Every time he applied for work he could truthfully say he had never been in jail. He was preacher-married to Mary, and had always done his best to provide for her and their two daughters. Now he was confused. Tribal memories welled up in his subconscious. Had he not somehow been outraged? His youngest daughter had just died trying to birth a fatherless child! The women could sense his bewilderment.

"Ah asked de Lawd for he'p, but sometimes—" Mattie's voice trailed off in quavering exhaustion.

"Ah'll make some coffee," Mary Jo said faintly, not wanting to go back in, but knowing what she must do.

"W'at mus' Ah do?" Joe asked, sitting down wearily on the steps.

"Go fo' de preachah w'en it's light," Mattie said. She leaned against the wall, and her sturdy shoulders shook in great, heaving sobs.

*   *   *   *   *

Mattie was tired, and she still had half a mile to walk to get home. The day was warm, and the sandy road, unpacked by any recent rain, was hard to walk in. Mattie slowed her gait, and eased her hundred and seventy pounds to a sitting position in front of the little Baptist church where she worshipped on Sundays. She plucked at the shapeless black dress to get the fresh air in, and wiped her broad face with a nondescript handkerchief.

Mattie was forty now, and the miles did not slip by so easily as they used to. A midwife did a lot of walking. In fact, so far as Mattie knew, no midwife had any other way of getting about. There were two doctors [who] lived about twenty miles away in the city. One of them drove a horse and buggy, and one had an automobile, but neither ventured this far from home very often. Mattie had seen Dr. Scott's automobile for the first time last month when—. She let the thought drift away. She had tried to keep from her mind the memories of that sad day when Joe had ridden twenty miles on a borrowed horse to get Dr. Scott to come and see little Mattie before they buried her. But the thought would come back now and then.

"Was dey anything Ah should have done, Doctah?" she had asked. Doctor Scott's answer had been kind, but Mattie had noticed a touch of frustration in it.

"No, Mattie, there was nothing you could have done—out here. Even in the hospital these things present difficulties. She wasn't far enough along. When she fell running like that—well, she broke the baby loose. Then nature called for it to be born right away, but her bones and muscles weren't ready, then he couldn't come. It wasn't your fault."

He wrote some more on the paper he had before him. "It wasn't your fault, that's true. But it isn't right—it isn't right."

He finished his writing. "I'll file this in the county seat. You can go ahead now."

Mattie took a deep breath. "Ain't much cash money in dese pahts, Doctah, but Joe got some mighty fine hams, and som' tatuhs."

The doctor's eyes crinkled. "Hickory smoked, too, I'll bet. Mattie, you've made a deal."

And then later, after he had cranked the car and moved the levers to diminish the roar. "Mattie, if you've got one coming along and you think she's going to have trouble, get her into town somehow and let me see her. I won't charge if she hasn't any money."

Mattie was thinking about this now as she rested. New ideas did not come easily, but she realized that this was something new. The white doctor had spoken to her as a sort of ally, as if they were somehow working together. It was the first time she had ever spoken with the doctor.

She wished Dr. Scott might have seen the fine girl baby she had delivered today. That was the third since—. Well, three alive in a row, that was pretty good. Mattie wanted to catch them all alive and healthy, but she never got past six or seven, and then would come a bad day, and her heart would be heavy.

Her eyes were closed. She opened them as she heard a footstep, and saw Preacher Smith coming toward her.

"Evenin', Pahson," Mattie said.

"Good evenin', Sistuh Morgan, Ah hope the Lawd has prospered you this day. Ah suppose you have been in attendance upon Sistuh Williams. And what was the Lawd's will this time?" The tall handsome carpenter set his lunch bucket down and peered at Mattie through gold-rimmed spectacles.

"A fine new sistuh fo' de congregation, but needin' a few yeahs to grow before she can say Amen," Mattie said, with a twinkle.

"Praise the Lawd—give thanks to the Almighty." His voice was booming now, and the spirit was upon him. "We thank Thee, Lawd, for Thy abundant mercy. We thank Thee for ca'yin' Sistuh Williams through the Valley of Death, and givin' into huh keepin' a little soul, fresh from Thy Presence. Oh, Lawd, grant that this child may live to grow in wisdom and statue, and learn to praise Thee all her days. We praise Thee, oh Lawd and give Thee thanks."

"Amen," Mattie breathed fervently. She could easily have burst out with the soprano obligatto of "All Praise the Power," for the eloquence of this righteous man always stimulated her to rapture, but she only sat breathless, enjoying the elation of the moment.

The pastor was still standing, gazing toward the sky. His Amen, his flock knew, was not the end of his communion. They had learned to wait patiently until the spirit released him. Suddenly he sat down wearily.

"Ovahhead. Ev'ry nail I driv today was ovahhead. Whuff."

"Ev'ry baby I 'livered today was stoop, stoop, stoop."

"Ah driv a *heap* o' nails."

"You only buildin' one house."

The man's merry laughter boomed in the quiet grove, and warmed Mattie's heart. They loved to tease each other. Though the Rev. Eustis Longfellow Smith could read and write, and wore shoes all the time, their stations in life were not too far apart. Both were quick witted, and they had a warm affection for each other.

"Ah'll go ovah and see Sistuh Williams tonight," he said. "Have they choosed a name?"

"Ah dunno. Didn't mention it," Mattie said.

"Well, Ah hope dey don't name huh fo' you like so many does. You got enough namesakes in the flock now." Mattie knew he meant it as a barb, but her mind was on something else.

"Preachuh," she spoke softly. "You asked me what was de Lawd's will. Ah'm askin' you de same. You reckon it's de Lawd's will w'en Ah catches one dead?"

His ebony face sombered. His eyes took on a far-away look. Those close to him knew this look. They would wait while he searched his soul for a revelation.

"No, Mattie," he said at last. "A merciful Lawd couldn't wish no such thing. But the Good Book tells us that trouble is sent to us to teach us something—to try our souls—to make us strong. We mus' puhsevere in tribulation."

Mattie knew the man was pontiffically [*sic*] correct, but she also knew the man. She looked at him side-long.

"Dat's de onliest answuh I know, Mattie. Dat's all I know," he said. They both knew it wasn't enough.

Their mood was shattered by the shrill call of Elva, the pastor's wife, from the little house adjoining the church.

"Mattie, is dat you down dere with Eustis? You come an' have suppah with us. We got 'gatuh tail."

Mattie sprang to her feet. "Elva, you is singin' lak an angel from Hebb'n," she shouted. Then to the parson, "Wheah you get 'gatuh tail?"

"From a 'gatuh."

*   *   *   *   *

A tiny shaft of sunlight poked Mattie in the eye and she awoke. The room was dark, its sashless windows shuttered against the night. She closed the shutters tightly every night of the year. They served to keep out cold—if any—insects, prowlers, and the "vapors," a night enemy known to her ancestors only after they had adopted some of the ways of their white masters. Mattie sat up and reached behind her to open the window above her bed.

The last few foraging roaches scurried for the darkness as Mattie pulled a greasy brown dress over her head. Her morning toilet thus completed, she shuffled to the stove, dropped in some small pieces of pine stump and a wad of paper, and set the mass afire with a match. A few more pieces of jack oak and the fire was ready to heat the oven for biscuits.

Then Mattie was ready for a daily ritual which she had not missed in many years. She wet her finger, stuch [*sic*] it in the ashes under the stove, and made a solid black smear across the date, Saturday, April 10, on the gigantic calendar on the wall of her room.

Some years ago, Mattie had found a tightly rolled sheet of paper that she suspected had fallen out of the mailman's buggy. Upon opening it, she had discovered a set of twelve beautiful pictures with what she knew were blocks of numbers printed below them. Eustis Smith had just come back from being ordained at Orlando, and she had shown it to him.

Ever since then Mattie had made it a project to get herself a new calendar, and have it ready to install in its place of honor one week after Christmas. Like many of her illiterate peers she could count in cardinal and ordinal numbers up to a dozen or so, and with a little coaching she had expanded this ability to include all the numbers under 32. Now she knew how to use her calendar to predict fairly closely when she would be needed by one of her prospective clients. Each was known by a mark of some sort, and Mattie's memory was acute enough that once a certain mark had been established in her mind as representing a certain client, it was not forgotten until it had served its purpose.

Her agile mind had had little trouble with the problem of changing calendars each year. The torn off pages were preserved, and the marks shifted over to the new pages when another calendar went into use. Mattie was not one to let the details of her business get out of hand.

Mattie stirred up her biscuits and det [sic] them to raise while she went out to see what worthwhile efforts her hands had made since her last inspection. She counted the eight birds pecking about in the yard, and carried the five fresh eggs into the house. Eight good hard-working hens and a rooster she had, and not a one had been stolen in nearly a year. That was because she had fortunately acquired the reputation of being a light sleeper, and of keeping a heavy hoe on the floor beside her bed, ready for action. Sometime back a non-working member of the community had gone about with a bandaged head for several days, claiming to have struck a tree branch while riding a horse. Rumor had it, however, that there was some vague connection between the wound and the hollering and cussing that had been heard around Mattie's chicken house. Anyway, her count remained at a satisfactory eight month after month.

That story, recalled occasionally with wry smiles, was attached firmly in the minds of older folks with one which had no humor in it. As they remembered it, Mattie had come home late one night and found a man waiting for her in her house. The two had been known to be casual friends, and Mattie was said by some to have acted as though she were willing for the relationship to progress. No one knew the details, but the man was found the next day where he had crawled some distance from Mattie's house, so battered that it appeared he might not make it. He did, but from then on no man, and very few women, bothered to ask Mattie why she remained unmarried.

And so she had remained, living alone in her untidy little house next to the Parkers, serving her community as midwife, working her garden patch, helping Joe with his pigs, and making barbeque for the white folks whenever they asked her. This was her chief source of cash income for few indeed were the clients who could pay in cash for her midwife services.

Mattie added some wood to the fire, and set her biscuits in the oven. A slice of ham and two of the eggs would be fried, and she would make a pot of coffee. Breakfast was a substantial meal with Mattie's people. Lunch was a word they did not know, and supper was again as heavy a meal as could be contrived. Fortunate was the family which had an older member not too feeble to spend the day fishing.

Mattie put the skillet on the stove and went over to examine her meager wardrobe. There was a barbeque tonight, and the white ladies had told Mattie that she must wear a clean white dress, and shoes, and a cap. Mattie knew what clean meant, and knew that it meant she would have to wash today. She glanced out in the yard. The boiler was there, and plenty of wood. There was home made lye soap in the box in the corner, so she was all set.

She glanced down at the shoes on the floor. Two pair were there. Her go-to-meetin' shoes, men's low cut Oxford style size 9, and her comfortable shoes, also originally made for a man, but adapted by wear, time and attrition to Mattie's needs. Possibly size 9 originally, they had long since burst out at the sole seams, and their ankle-hugging uppers were sturdy and dependable. These would have to do for the barbeque. The others were for church and that was that.

Then came the bright spot in Mattie's morning. Mattie dreaded washing and ironing like she dreaded a breech delivery. But her salvation was at hand. She heard Mary Jo's voice at the door.

"Aunt Mattie, you gotta bahb'cue tonight. You want me to wash an' iron your dress an' apron?"

"You do dat an' Ah'll give you a nickel, chile," said Mattie, trying to keep the rapture from her voice.

Mary Jo came in and took the dress from the peg. "Wheah's de apron?"

"Undah de bed, Ah reckon," Mattie's tone implied that the girl should know where to find the apron.

Mary Jo, her own dress spotless, fished the mess from its dark hiding place. Roaches showered from its folds and scurried away. The gingham mass gave off the almost physical odor of an ancient abbatoir.

"Aunt Mat-tie!"

The apron was doomed. Mattie could see that. Mary Jo carried it across the room between thumb and forefinger and stuffed it in the stove.

"Ah'll len' you one of Mama's fo' tonight, Aunt Mattie." Her face brightened. "An' den you buy me some gingum and Ah'll make you a new one on Miz' Smith's sewin' machine."

"All right, honey." She watched the joy of her heart run swiftly across the yard, white dress flying behind her.

Mattie dropped a slice of ham into the skillet, noting the satisfying sizzle and aroma that erupted from it. Then she went to check her finances. From behind a loose brick in the chimney she took a rag which had been tied in a tight knot. From this she extracted her liquid assets. There was a whole dollar, tightly balled, and a quarter and two dimes. That was good. Many a family in the community did not see that much cash in a whole week. Some did better, of course. Some men worked steady for fifty cents a day. Well, she was as good as any man when it came to earning money. She would get fifty cents tonight for just six or seven hours work at the barbeque. What was fifteen cents for apron money every year or so. Besides, she needed the apron for her midwifery, too.

Mattie finished her breakfast with the tenth biscuit and fourth cup of coffee. She was replete now, and she felt good. She tossed the ham bone, biscuit crumbs, coffee grounds, and a handful of corn to the chickens, and hung the skillet on its peg. She wiped the plate vigorously with a rag, and threw the rag in the fireplace. Then she shuffled to the porch and sat down in her rocker. The world was warm around her. The amaryllis was audaciously pink. The red bud and dogwood waved their blossoms at the naked pecans, and little white baby clouds nestled in invisible angels' arms across the sky. A mockingnerd [*sic*] poked bits of worm into the cavernous beaks of her butterbean-sized young. Mattie leaned back and hummed softly as her eyes began to close. Mary Jo's industrious splashings could be heard in the next yard. A nickel was a lot of money, but then—Mattie could afford it. There would be good barbeque—her own barbeque—made with the white folks' ingredients—that she would eat until her eyes bugged—after the white folks were through—somebody plowing over there—Mary Jo washing—younguns scrapping—everybody busy— happy—praise the Lord for his Goodness—this was a good day, this Saturday, April 10, 1910.

*   *   *   *   *

A truly comprehensive history of the program for the control and education of Florida's midwives cannot be written. A large percentage of the material that would be needed for such an effort went into the waste baskets of officials long since retired or passed from this scene. That which remains is fragmentary, but the fragments together add up to a sizeable volume. Some of the material is apocryphal from the strictly official point of view, but it is revealing, and adds salt and pepper to the meat and potatoes of our story. Its flavor will be found in the fictional parts of the work.

Before venturing far into our review it would be well to have a definition of terms. We shall accept as established the premise that any person who assists a woman in childbirth can be called a midwife for the moment. But our focus will be upon a somewhat more strict interpretation of the word. We shall use the term *midwife* to apply to that person who by choice or circumstance is set up in the community as one to be called upon regularly or habitually to assist in human birth. This person may be man or woman of any race. Let it be clear, however, that the word *midwife* alone carries no implication of any special knowledge, training or authorization except that which might be acquired by experience—as one who has learned to swim after a fashion by thrashing about to keep from drowning.

It might also be well to define for the unfamiliar the comparison between the ignorant, superstitious midwife and the quack. The distance between them is infinite. While the quack acts in his own interests for whatever he may gain from it, the midwife can only be considered as trying to help others. Her practice, however pleasant or difficult it may have been, was something other than lucrative. Only during the last very few years have a few midwives found themselves in the situation of making what could be called at best a meager living from their practice.

One more bit of clarification should be set forth here. Our history, that portion of our work which constitutes the final section of each chapter, will be that of the midwife control and education program of the Florida State Board of Health, not the history of the midwives themselves. The latter, though more exotic than statistical tables, exists only in remembered anecdote, and hardly lends itself to serious compilation for any worthy purpose.

Midwives may be assumed to have been part of the Florida scene since the first Apalachee [Seminole crossed out] or Timuquan baby gasped its first breath on the peninsula. The early conquerors and settlers had doctors with them, but these worthies' time and talents were strained to their limits by such anomalies as the wounds of the military and the governor's gout, and scant indeed was the attention given to ordinary childbirth. In fact, it is within the memory of living man that pregnancy was raised above the status of a good case of *grippe* and began to call for the attention of a physician—among those who could afford this luxury. Here was work for the midwife.

The greatest factor, however, in the growth of Florida's midwife problem, was the presence of a large and prolific secondary population, only recently released from slavery—a move regarded by many as more lateral than vertical—uneducated, superstitious, and forced by economic circumstance if not by choice to live in their own socially isolated communities under the poorest conditions of sanitation and asepsis. It is estimated that an extremely large proportion of these people, male and female, lived out their lives without ever seeing a doctor of medicine face to face.

In the early spring of 1910, when Little Mattie died of her miscarriage, the history of the midwifery program in Florida had not yet begun. The word *midwife* had appeared once only in the official records of the State Board of Health (Florida Health Notes, Annual Reports, and other papers), and that was in a side reference made in 1901 in his annual report to the State Health

Officer, Dr. Joseph Y. Porter, by Dr. J. M. Abbot, of Pasco County. While refer-ring to the prevalence of certain diseases in his district during the year, he wrote: "—and some cases of puerperal fever, as the midwives attend to about all such cases (in this area) as elsewhere, so it is only in desperate cases, or as a last resort, that the medical fraternity are called in. I think midwives should be taught asepsis, but I have never met one yet who did not know more than all the obstetricians in the world, and I do not see how they can be taught, for they would astonish the wisdom of this mundane globe."

While it is not difficult to imagine a sizeable group of colleagues disagreeing with Dr. Abbot's conclusions, it is easy to surmise that he was not the only advocate of education for the midwives. The aggressive and progressive Dr. Porter is said to have favored the idea, but the records do not mention it until later. Midwives, in Florida in 1910, went about their affairs as had their prede-cessors since time immemorial, unhampered and unaided.

Notes

Preface

1. Carrol Smith Rosenberg, "The Female World of Love and Ritual: Relations Between Women in Nineteenth-Century America," *Signs* 1, no. 1 (Autumn 1975): 1–29.
2. Jane B. Donegan, *Women and Men Midwives: Medicine, Morality, and Misogyny in Early America* (Westport, Conn.: Greenwood Press, 1978); Judy Barrett Litoff, *American Midwives, 1860 to the Present* (Westport, Conn.: Greenwood Press, 1978).

Introduction

1. The White House Conference on Child Health and Protection, a November 1930 conference attended by over three thousand people, was assembled by the Hoover administration and enlisted twelve hundred experts to do preparatory research for sixteen months. The Committee on the Costs of Medical Care was a five-year study organized in May 1927 by leaders in medicine, public health, and the social sciences. And the New York Academy of Medicine's Committee on Public Health Relations conducted a three-year study of maternal deaths in the city beginning in January 1930.
2. White House Conference on Child Health and Protection, *Obstetric Education* (New York, 1932), 216–17, as cited in Litoff, *American Midwives,* 109.
3. Sam Shapiro, Edward R. Schlesinger, and Robert E. L. Nesbitt, Jr., *Infant, Perinatal, Maternal, and Childbirth Morbidity in the United States*

(Cambridge, Mass., 1968); *White House Conference on Child Health and Protection, 1930: Addresses and Abstracts of Committee Reports* (New York, 1931); Bureau of the Census, *Vital Statistics of the United States, 1970* (Washington, D.C., 1974); White House Conference on Child Health and Protection, *Fetal, Newborn, and Maternal Morbidity and Mortality* (New York, 1933); Ransom S. Hooker, *Maternal Mortality in New York City: A Study of All Puerperal Deaths, 1930–1932* (New York, 1933); and George W. Kosmak, "Certain Aspects of the Midwife Problem in Relation to the Medical Profession and Community," *Medical Record* 85 (June 1914). All statistical information in this paragraph is cited in Litoff, *American Midwives*, 108–11.

4. Litoff, *American Midwives*, 18–24.

5. This is a statement made by Dr. Joseph B. De Lee, founder of Chicago Lying-in Hospital in 1895 and a leader of the movement to eradicate the midwife. Joseph B. De Lee, "Report of Sub-Committee for Illinois," *Transactions of the American Association for the Study and Prevention of Infant Mortality* 5 (1914): 231; Joseph B. De Lee, "Progress Toward Ideal Obstetrics," *Transactions of the American Association for the Study and Prevention of Infant Mortality* 6 (1915): 117. These are cited in Litoff, *American Midwives*, 67.

6. John F. Moran, "The Endowment of Motherhood," *Journal of the American Medical Association* 64 (January 1915): 125–26, as cited in Litoff, *American Midwives*, 69.

7. Richard W. Wertz and Dorothy C. Wertz, *Lying-In: A History of Childbirth in America* (New York: Free Press, 1977), 216.

8. Olivia Dunbar, "To the Baby, Debtor," *Good Housekeeping*, November 1918, 35; S. Josephine Baker, "Getting the Right Start," *Ladies' Home Journal*, August 1930, 80; Carolyn Conant Van Blascom, "Rat Pie among the Black Midwives," *Harper's*, February 1930, 322–27.

9. Wertz and Wertz, *Lying-In*, 151.

10. William R. Nicholson, "The Midwife Situation," *Transactions of the American Gynecological Society* 42 (1917): 623, as cited in Litoff, *American Midwives*, 77.

11. A white nurse offended Mrs. Black with this statement after her rapid birth at the hospital. See interview with Jenny Black, p. 105.

12. Neal Devitt, "The Statistical Case for Elimination of the Midwife: Fact versus Prejudice, 1890–1935," part 1, *Women and Health* 4 (Spring 1979): 82.

13. Speech by Ethel J. Kirkland, a Florida public health nursing consultant, made in Jacksonville, Florida, in October 1973, in memory of Jule O. Graves. Copy to be filed with the University of Florida Nursing Program and given to me by Iona Pettengill, senior community health nursing consultant with HRS.

14. From the preface to "Midwifery in Florida," in State Board of Health, the Midwifery Files, 1924–1961 (with emphasis on 1930s and 1940s), series 904, boxes 1–8, Florida State Archives, Tallahassee (hereafter cited as FSA).

Chapter One. Charismatic Leader: The Community's View of the Midwife

1. Evelyn Reynolds, interview with author.

2. Many mothers named their babies after the attending midwife.

3. At the June 1984 Southern "Granny" Midwives Conference, held at Spelman College in Atlanta, Georgia, there was discussion about the use of the term *granny*. Some believed the designation was of slave origin and, for that reason, should be replaced with the word *traditional*. Both terms will be used here interchangeably.

4. Mary Keller, interview with author.

5. The older rural midwives refer to delivering babies as "catching" babies, reflective of their noninterventive perspective on childbirth. It is the *mothers* that deliver the babies.

6. Evelyn Reynolds, interview with author.

7. For a period in Florida's history, the office through which midwives' licenses were granted was headquartered in Jacksonville.

8. Johnnie Seeley, interview with author.

9. "The board" is a term the midwives used to refer to the midwifery advisory board, a state agency that granted or denied licenses to practice mid-

test238   Notes

wifery. See chap. 2 for the history of the Florida State Board of Health's
role in midwifery.

10. David Stewart, "Skillful Midwifery: The Highest and Safest Standard," in
The Five Standards for Safe Childbearing: Good Nutrition, Skillful Midwifery, Natural Childbirth, Home Birth, Breastfeeding, ed. David Stewart
(Marble Hill, Mo.: NAPSAC International, 1981), 142.

11. Arthur F. Raper, *Tenants of the Almighty* (New York: Macmillan, 1943),
299–300.

12. Mary Beth Chambers, interview with author.

13. Gertha Couric, "Midwives Are Called Granny," in Federal Writer's Project, Papers of the Regional Director William Terry Couch, Southern Historical Collection, University of North Carolina, Chapel Hill.

14. James Seay Brown, Jr., *Up Before Daylight: Life Histories from the Alabama Writer's Project, 1938–1939* (Tuscaloosa: University of Alabama
Press, 1982), 133.

15. Karen Cox, "Midwives and Granny Women," in *Foxfire 2*, ed. Eliot Wigginton (Garden City, N.Y.: Anchor Press, 1973), 288.

16. Jenny Black, interview with author, August 5, 1981.

17. Augusta Wilson, interview with author, August 6, 1981.

18. Ibid.

19. Rosalind Stephenson, interview with author.

20. Ibid.

21. Mary Lee Jones, interview with author.

22. K. C. Cole, *What Only a Mother Can Tell You about Having a Baby* (New
York: Berkley Publishing Corp., 1980), 218.

23. Cole, *What Only a Mother Can Tell*, 68–69.

24. Rosalind Stephenson, interview with author.

25. Cole, *What Only a Mother Can Tell*, 253.

26. Mary Keller, interview with author.

27. Mary Beth Chambers, interview with author.

28. Evelyn Reynolds, interview with author.

29. Rosalind Stephenson, interview with author.

30. Ibid.

31. Emma Newton, interview with author. Mrs. Newton is an eighty-four-

year-old white midwife residing in the Appalachian Mountains of Tennessee.
32. While interviewing, circumstances were not always conducive to using a tape recorder. For these I took what notes I could. Mrs. MacBride had granted me an interview on one occasion without the recorder but canceled our second appointment, fearful of repercussions from the local county health department. Rev. Brown is a busy pastor, and I considered myself lucky to pass what time I could with her on the front lawn of her church.
33. Cox, "Midwives and Granny Women," 282.
34. Ibid, 284.
35. Emma Newton, interview with author.

Chapter Two. Public Health Menace: The State's View of the Midwife

1. The Sheppard-Towner Maternity and Infancy Protection Act of 1921 provided for "instruction in the hygiene of maternity and infancy through public-health nurses, visiting nurses, consultation centers, child-care conferences, and literature distribution." The American Medical Association and state medical societies actively lobbied against it. From its six-year appropriations of $7,680,000, programs for the training and control of midwives were instituted in all but three states.
2. These statistics are cited in the files of the state supervisor of midwives Joyce Ely, series 904, box 1, FSA.
3. In Florida records, there are three different estimates of the number of midwives practicing in Florida: Ethel Kirkland quoted a 1930 survey that found thirty-three hundred self-proclaimed midwives; Dolores Wennlund quoted four thousand midwives in 1931, and probably twice that many the Board of Health was not aware of, in her report entitled "The Florida Midwifery Dilemma"; and Joyce Ely estimated fifteen hundred midwives in 1933. The first two citations come from the files of Iona Pettengill,

series 904, box 1, and the last is from the 1933 minutes of a meeting of Florida health officials, series 904, box 1, FSA.

4. Statement made by Joyce Ely, RN, state supervisor of midwives, in minutes of 1933 meeting of state health officials, series 904, box 1, FSA.

5. This material comes from the following paragraph in "Midwifery in Florida," FSA:

> The dirt, ignorance and superstition of early midwifery will not be belabored in this work. Had they not existed as a serious problem no midwifery program would have been undertaken. Had they not been the prime reason for Florida's one-in-ten infant death rate they would not now have to be looked back upon as fortunately overcome, as were hog cholera, yellow fever, malaria, and other environmental vexations, which caused a visiting Pennsylvania doctor to write back to his family; "This is an inclement place, abounding in pestilence, and surely in summer a capital setting for Dante's Inferno."

6. Devitt, "Elimination of the Midwife," 89–90.

7. Wertz and Wertz, *Lying-In*, 125–28.

8. J. W. Williams, "Medical Education and the Midwife Problem in the United States, *Journal of the American Medical Association* 58 (1912): 1–7, as cited in Devitt, "Elimination of the Midwife," 84–85.

9. Harold Speert, *The Sloane Hospital Chronicle* (Philadelphia: 1963), 80, as cited in Litoff, *American Midwives*, 20.

10. White House Conference on Child Health and Protection, *Obstetric Education*, as cited in Devitt, "Elimination of the Midwife," 86.

11. Paul Coughlin, director of the Leon County Health Department, to Lucille J. Marsh, director of the Bureau of Maternal and Child Health, 3 August 1944, series 904, box 5, FSA.

12. Minutes of a 1933 meeting of state health officials, series 904, box 1, FSA.

13. T. J. Hill, "Some Remarks on the Midwifery Question: Must the Midwife Perish?" *Medical Record* 4 (October 1898): 475, as cited in Litoff, *American Midwives*, 103.

14. O. R. Thompson, "Midwife Problem," *Journal of the Medical Association of Georgia* 16 (April 1927): 136, as cited in Litoff, *American Midwives*, 78.

15. Statement made by Dr. Michael Moreton in his testimony against the new midwifery law before the Florida House of Representatives Committee on

Tourism and Economic Development, 12 February 1982. The statement was made in reference to creating a Board of Midwifery: "There is a great deal of voodoo medicine going on in South Florida with animal sacrifices and the like. And I wonder if—whether it is necessary for DPR [Department of Professional Regulation] to come up with a Board of Voodoo Medicine in order to make sure that the chickens have been slaughtered in quite the appropriate manner."

16. Preface to "A Long Dark Night: The Midwives of Florida," by David K. Fulton, series 904, box 1, FSA.

17. Minutes of a 1933 meeting of state health officials, series 904, box 1, FSA.

18. Ibid.

19. Ethel Kirkland, speech delivered in Jacksonville, Florida, October 1973, transcript, author's collection.

20. This information is gleaned from a program of this institute's opening ceremony, author's collection.

21. A midwife's bag was a black satchel in which the midwife carried the materials she needed when attending a birth. These were usually linens, gauze, string, and scissors, and silver nitrate for the baby's eyes. They were not to carry any kind of unauthorized drugs. The midwife was instructed to sterilize all contents as well as clean the bag after each birth. Health officials conducted bag inspections to check for compliance with this standard.

22. A miniature replica of this doll is among the midwifery files of the Florida State Board of Health collection, FSA, along with extensive correspondence on its patent.

23. Minutes of a 1933 meeting of state health officials, series 904, box 1, FSA.

24. The first mention of a midwife's manual in state records is of a 1923 twenty-page book that emphasized the cleanliness of midwife, patient, and home. It was a catechism on prenatal care, identifying emergency situations, and what to do in cases of hemorrhage and accidents of labor.

25. These slides were donated to the University of Florida School of Nursing in Gainesville, Florida. They are in the process of being catalogued. Negatives of the slides are housed at the Florida State Archives in Tallahassee, Florida.

26. Ruth Doran, public health nursing consultant, to Dr. Fred Mayes of the Children's Bureau in Atlanta, 13 November 1944, series 904, box 5, FSA.
27. "Plan for Improving the Midwife Service," 1944–1946, series 904, box 5, FSA.
28. Coughlin to Marsh, 3 August 1944, series 904, box 5, FSA.
29. Molly C. Dougherty, "Southern Lay Midwives as Ritual Specialists," in *Women in Ritual and Symbolic Roles,* ed. Judith Hoch-Smith and Anita Spring (New York: Plenum Press, 1978), 158–59.
30. Report on Public Health Nursing in the 1932 *Annual Reports of the State Board of Health of Florida* (Jacksonville).
31. Report on Public Health Nursing in the 1942 *Annual Reports of the State Board of Health of Florida* (Jacksonville). The distinction between a lay midwife and a nurse-midwife is one of training and recognition. The lay midwife had no formal education but learned her craft via the more empirical format of apprenticeship training. The nurse-midwife was a product of the modern medical system and was usually a registered nurse with specialized training in obstetrics. The nurse-midwife, receiving her education within the university model, had less of a noninterventive orientation than the lay midwife.
32. This refers to Mrs. Wilson's experience, as cited on p. 76. There was no oral or written record of the county's side on this matter. However, one health official recalled the reputation of the county nurse in charge of the case to be decidedly anti-midwife.
33. Report on Public Health Nursing in the 1966 *Annual Reports of the State Board of Health of Florida* (Jacksonville).

Chapter Three. The Uneasy Meeting of Tradition and State

1. Cox, "Midwives and Granny Women," 286.
2. J. Clifton Edgar, "The Education, Licensing, and Supervision of the Midwife," *Transactions of the American Association for the Study and Preven-*

tion of Infant Mortality 6 (1915): 92, 96–97, as cited in Litoff, *American Midwives,* 79.

3. S. W. Newmayer, "The Status of Midwifery in Pennsylvania and a Study of the Midwives in Philadelphia," *Monthly Cyclopedia and Medical Bulletin* 4 (1911): 713 and 718, as cited in Litoff, *American Midwives,* 80.

4. Jule O. Graves, "The Midwife Program in Florida," *Public Health Nursing* (October 1939).

5. Mary Beth Chambers, interview with author.

6. Escambia County Supervisor of Nurses to the state midwife consultant, letter, July 1944, series 904, box 5, FSA.

7. In the minutes of a 1933 meeting of Florida health officials (series 904, box 1, FSA,) Joyce Ely, state supervisor of midwives, reported that 483 new cases were recorded at the Jacksonville clinic for prenatal exams that year. Eighty percent of these were referred by midwives, and 138 cases opted to have their deliveries at the Brewster Colored Hospital.

8. Evelyn Reynolds, interview with author.

9. Tallahassee Memorial Regional Medical Center was involved with local controversies relative to their obstetric section. One of these concerned a request by the newly opened (1979) Tallahassee Community Hospital, a Hospital Corporation of America enterprise, to open a birthing facility. Their certificate of need, the first step in its application to open, was challenged. And after two years of appeals and counterappeals involving the state's Department of Health and Rehabilitative Services (HRS) and the district circuit court, the birthing center won its approval and opened in 1984, despite TMRMC opposition.

10. For example, two nurse midwives, who planned to open a delivery practice in Nashville and successfully secured emergency backup from a physician, were denied hospital privileges at three hospitals. The doctor involved also lost his malpractice insurance. *Wall Street Journal,* 22 February 1983.

11. This story remains unsubstantiated by either the midwife involved or county records. The former refused to discuss the matter, fearful of legal repercussions and/or unwilling to go into unpleasant past events. The information comes from the midwife's friend and former employee who

worked at the home during the inspections. Many interested people, including the midwife's minister, volunteered to talk with her, but she could not be persuaded to be interviewed. County records were said to have been destroyed to make room for more recent records.

12. Report on Public Health Nursing in the 1962 *Annual Reports of the State Board of Health of Florida.*
13. Rosalind Stephenson, interview with author.
14. Johnnie Seeley, interview with author.
15. Mary Beth Chambers, interview with author.
16. Evelyn Reynolds, interview with author.
17. Jule O. Graves played an active part in Florida's public health programs for twenty years beginning in 1926. She worked with the Seminole Indians, traveling alone deep into the Everglades. And she developed "Miss Chase," the obstetrical mannequin used for the instruction of midwives. Her lifetime dedication to public health and humanitarian endeavors are lauded throughout Florida State Board of Health records.
18. Mary Lee Jones, interview with author.
19. Rosalind Stephenson, interview with author.
20. Ina May Gaskin, *Spiritual Midwifery* (Summertown, Tenn.: Book Publishing Co., 1978), 11.
21. In 1972 the Public Health Nursing Advisory Committee, the county nursing directors, the Florida Association of County Health Officers, and the director of the Division of Health had all publicly called for the total phaseout of the lay midwifery program. Nurse-midwives were part of the medical community and thus shared the perspective of most medical professionals. Efforts to bridge this gap between nurse-midwives and lay midwives were made by lay midwife proponents. The public health administration's attempts to keep these two types of midwives on opposite sides of the issue were successful, although the nurse-midwives are increasingly open to communication between the two.
22. Dolores Wennlund, appendix A-1 to "The Issue: Midwifery," Florida HRS, Health Program Office, n.d. This report outlines the progress of the state's midwifery program up through the 1970s.
23. Ibid, appendix A-2.

24. Apgar scores rate the newborn's respiration, skin tone, color, and other vital indications on a ten-point scale, zero representing a stillborn. The birth attendant evaluates these vital signs at one minute after birth and again at five minutes. One HRS official reported that a few of the older midwives had inserted a zero Apgar rating for healthy babies.
25. Rosalind Stephenson, interview with author.
26. Mary Lee Jones, interview with author.
27. Ibid.

Chapter Four. A Rebirth of American Midwifery

1. Interview with a thirty-year-old white midwife.
2. Along with the interviews of the older women, I interviewed young midwives and their clients as well.
3. Gerda Lerner, *The Majority Finds Its Past: Placing Women in History* (New York: Oxford University Press, 1979), 146–50.
4. Mary Keller, interview with author.

Selected Bibliography

Arms, Suzanne. *Immaculate Deception: A New Look at Women and Child-birth in America.* Boston: Houghton Mifflin, 1975.

Brown, James Seay, Jr. *Up Before Daylight: Life Histories from the Alabama Writer's Project, 1938–1939.* Tuscaloosa: University of Alabama Press, 1982.

Campbell, Marie. *Folks Do Get Born.* New York: Rinehart and Co., 1946.

Cole, K. C. *What Only a Mother Can Tell You about Having a Baby.* New York: Berkley Publishing Corp., 1981.

Couric, Gertha. "Midwives Are Called Granny." Papers of the Federal Writer's Project Regional Director William Terry Couch. Southern Historical Collection. University of North Carolina, Chapel Hill.

Cox, Karen. "Midwives and Granny Women." In *Foxfire 2,* edited by Eliot Wigginton. Garden City, N.Y.: Anchor Press, 1973.

De Lee, Joseph B. "The Prophylactic Forceps Operation." *American Journal of Obstetrics and Gynecology* 1 (1920): 34–44.

Devitt, Neal. "The Statistical Case for Elimination of the Midwife: Fact versus Prejudice, 1890–1935." *Women and Health* 4 (Spring, Summer 1979): 81–96, 169–86.

Donegan, Jane B. *Women and Men Midwives: Medicine, Morality, and Misogyny in Early America.* Westport, Conn.: Greenwood Press, 1978.

Dougherty, Molly C. "Southern Lay Midwives as Ritual Specialists." In *Women in Ritual and Symbolic Roles,* edited by Judith Hoch-Smith and Anita Spring. New York: Plenum Press, 1978.

Dye, Nancy Schrom. "Mary Breckinridge, the Frontier Nursing Service, and the Introduction of Nurse-Midwifery in the United States." *Bulletin of the History of Medicine* 57 (1983): 485–507.

Ehrenreich, Barbara, and Deirdre English. *Witches, Midwives, and Nurses: A*

History of Women Healers. Old Westbury, N.Y.: The Feminist Press, 1973.
———. *For Her Own Good: 150 Years of Experts' Advice to Women.* Garden City, N.Y.: Anchor Press, 1978.
Gaskin, Ina May. *Spiritual Midwifery.* Summertown, Tenn.: Book Publishing Co., 1978.
Graham, Harvey. *Eternal Eve: The History of Gynecology and Obstetrics.* New York: Doubleday, 1951.
Holmes, Linda P. "Alabama Granny Midwife." *Journal of the Medical Society of New Jersey* 81 (May 1984): 389–91.
Kirkland, Ethel J. "Memory Jewels of Jule O. Graves." Speech delivered at conference of directors of the Florida Public Health Association, Inc., Jacksonville, Florida, October 1973.
Kitzinger, Sheila. *Women As Mothers.* New York: Random House, 1980.
Kobrin, Francis E. "The American Midwife Controversy: A Crisis in Professionalization." *Bulletin of the History of Medicine* 40 (1966): 350–63.
Leavitt, Judith Walzer. " 'Science' Enters the Birthing Room." *Journal of American History* 70 (1983): 281–305.
Leavitt, Judith Walzer, and Whitney Walton. " 'Down to Death's Door': Women's Perceptions of Childbirth in America." In *Women and Health in America: Historical Readings,* edited by Judith Walzer Leavitt. University of Wisconsin Press, 1984.
Lerner, Gerda. *The Majority Finds Its Past: Placing Women in History.* New York: Oxford University Press, 1979.
Litoff, Judith Barrett. *The American Midwife Debate.* Westport, Conn.: Greenwood Press, 1986.
———. *American Midwives, 1860 to the Present.* Westport, Conn.: Greenwood Press, 1978.
Lubic, Ruth Watson. "The Politics of Childbirth Today." In *Second Motherhood Symposium Proceedings.* Women's Studies Research Center: University of Wisconsin at Madison, 1982.
Nihell, Elizabeth. *A Treatise on the Art of Midwifery: Setting Forth Various Abuses Therein, Especially as to the Practice with Instruments.* London, 1760.
Raper, Arthur F. *Tenants of the Almighty.* New York: Macmillan, 1943.

Rich, Adrienne. *Of Woman Born.* New York: Norton, 1976.

Rosenberg, Carrol Smith. "The Female World of Love and Ritual: Relations Between Women in Nineteenth-Century America." *Signs* 1, no. 1 (Autumn 1975): 1–29.

Sablosky, Ann H. "The Power of the Forceps: A Comparative Analysis of the Midwife Historically and Today." *Women and Health,* January–February 1976, 10–13.

State Board of Health. The Midwifery Files, 1924–1961 (with emphasis on 1930s and 1940s), series 904, boxes 1–8, Florida State Archives, Tallahassee.

Stewart, David. "Skillful Midwifery: The Highest and Safest Standard." In *The Five Standards for Safe Childbearing: Good Nutrition, Skillful Midwifery, Natural Childbirth, Home Birth, Breastfeeding,* edited by David Stewart. Marble Hill, Mo.: NAPSAC International, 1981.

Walsh, Mary Roth. *Doctors Wanted: No Women Need Apply: Sexual Barriers in the Medical Profession, 1835–1975.* New Haven: Yale University Press, 1977.

Wennlund, Dolores M. "The Issue: Midwifery." Florida Department of Health and Rehabilitative Services, Health Program Office, n.d.

Wertz, Richard W., and Dorothy C. Wertz. *Lying-In: A History of Childbirth in America.* New York: Free Press, 1977.

Women's Cooperative Guild. *Maternity: Letters from Working Women.* London: G. Beu and Sons, 1915.

Young, Patrick. "The Thoroughly Modern Midwife." *Saturday Review,* September 1972, 42–43.

Index

Abortion, 30–31, 61
Africa, 5
Apprenticeship training, 10, 12,
    18–19, 63, 66, 67, 101, 123, 140,
    142, 148–49, 167, 169–70,
    174–75, 176, 180, 193, 204,
    206–7, 211
Asepsis, 38, 42, 233

Birth attendants, 16–17, 19–20,
    22–23, 77, 108, 109–10,
    117–37, 153–54, 184, 186–87,
    219–20
Birthing mannequin, 42, 244
Breastfeeding, 80–81, 85, 163, 187
Bureau of Education and Child
    Welfare, 34

California, 60
The Calling, 13–16, 33, 46, 68, 137,
    148–50, 166, 169, 180, 213
Chamberlen, Peter, 4
Channing, Walter, 3
Chase, Miss (birthing mannequin), 42,
    244
Childbed fever, 1, 3, 38

Committee on the Costs of Medical
    Care, 1–2, 235 (n. 1)
Confinement period, 21–22, 152,
    160–61, 162–63, 165–66, 194
Coughlin, Paul, 45

Dixon, Sallie, 18
Doctor's permit, 46, 53–55, 56, 91,
    95, 141, 147, 168, 175–76

Edgar, J. Clifton, 50
Educational programs for midwives,
    3, 34–35, 39, 41, 43, 44–46, 49,
    63–64, 66, 99, 220
Ely, Joyce, 40–41
England, 2
European midwives, 2–3, 7, 139

The Farm, 60–61
Fees, 28–29, 46–47, 59, 87, 147,
    152, 169, 174, 191, 199, 200, 214
Florida Agricultural and Mechanical
    College, 42, 44, 220
Florida Department of Health and
    Rehabilitative Services, 53, 60, 62,
    64, 204

Florida Department of Professional Regulation, 64
Florida State Board of Health, 11, 18, 34, 37, 47, 48, 51, 57

Gadsden County, Florida, 55
Georgia, 27, 55, 138, 142, 150, 159, 168, 170, 204
Graves, Jule O., viii, 42, 58, 244 (n. 17)

Hanson, Henry, 41
Hill, T. J., 40
Hinson, Alberta, 18
Holmes, Oliver Wendell, 3
Home-birth movement, 56, 60–64, 66, 67, 70–72, 88, 155
Hospital birth, 1, 18, 77–79, 80, 101, 102–5, 134, 135

Immigration laws, 7
Infant and maternal mortality rates, 1–3, 37–38, 41, 80, 87–88, 98, 141, 172, 178

Jackson County, Florida, 55
Jacksonville, Florida, 123, 169, 176, 203, 215
Jones, Janie, 53

Kirkland, Ethel, 41, 43
Knox, J. H. Mason, 2

Leon County, Florida, 55
Liberty County, Florida, 55

License revocations, 20, 49, 58, 73, 76, 190, 200
Licensing of midwifery, 34–35, 47–49, 50–51, 62, 65, 67, 145, 149, 169, 170, 179, 198, 207, 209

Macon, Georgia, 40
Malpractice suits, 65–66, 173, 175, 178, 201, 206, 215
Marsh (doctor), 53
Maryland State Bureau of Child Hygiene, 2
Maternity homes, 27–28, 56, 82, 88–89, 91–95, 100, 166, 171, 190–91
Miami, Florida, 53
Midwife certificate, 42–43
Midwife clubs, 45–46, 51, 179, 195, 198, 208, 209–10, 215
Midwife institutes, 42–43, 174, 220–21
Midwifery laws: in 1931, 34, 40, 44, 47, 48, 53, 62; in 1982, 40, 60–67, 124, 143, 146, 201, 203–5, 214–15; in 1984, 67
Midwife's bag, 43, 45, 46, 215, 241 (n. 21)
Midwives, traditional: history of, xiii–ix, 72; as "ignorant, dirty, and superstitious," 4–7, 36, 39–40; and clients, 5, 6, 99–100, 102–16, 154–55, 159–66; and family involvement, 10, 24, 27–28, 84–85, 88–90; in family trade,

10–12, 15, 16, 17, 86–88, 123, 148, 167, 169, 180–81, 184, 187, 197, 208, 217; and religion, 13, 19, 20, 22, 32, 76, 110, 149–50, 154, 192, 212; bedside manner of, 19–21, 26, 75–76, 131, 150, 156, 177, 183, 185, 187, 192, 196, 211, 217–19; and "illegitimate" children, 30, 82
Moreton, Michael, 241 (n. 15)
Multiple births, 29–30, 130–31, 141, 182, 201, 221–22

New Jersey, 187, 191
Newmayer, S. W., 51
New York, 50
New York Academy of Medicine's Committee on Public Health Relations, 12, 235–36 (n. 1)
Nurse-midwives, 41, 47–48, 51, 62, 63, 66, 67, 124, 158, 181, 220, 242 (n. 31), 244 (n. 10), 245 (n. 21)
Nurse Training Act (1975), 62

Obstetrics, 3–4, 12, 71; operative intervention, 1, 3, 4–5, 6, 38, 64, 75; schools of, 1, 4, 38–39; and economic competition with midwives, 4, 7, 47, 48, 127, 171, 200, 214

Pennsylvania, 38
Pensacola, Florida, 53
Phase-out of midwifery, 6–7, 8, 41,

43, 48–49, 50–57, 58–60, 74, 86, 87, 90–92, 94, 97–99, 142, 167–68, 170, 172, 174, 188–89, 197, 200, 245 (n. 21)
Preparations for birth, 74, 75, 87, 151, 156, 164, 177, 206
county, Public health supervision, 45–46, 48–49, 51, 52, 58–59, 63–66, 87, 141, 144–45, 146–47, 156–57, 171, 172, 200, 203–5, 215–16
Puerperal fever, 1, 3, 38

Retirement of midwives, 47, 51–52, 137, 138–39, 144–46

Semmelweis, Ignaz, 3
Shelby, Mary Etta, 53
Sheppard-Towner Maternity and Infancy Protection Act (1921), 35, 239 (n. 1)
Silver nitrate, 4, 35
Sims, J. Marion, 4
State supervision of midwifery, 34, 43, 45–46, 48, 63
Stearns, John, 3
Summertown, Tennessee, 60

Tallahassee, Florida, 42, 44, 55, 64, 142
Tampa, Florida, 40, 62
Tennessee, 29, 60, 192
Thompson, O. R., 40

U.S. Children's Bureau, 44

Welfare and government assistance,
53, 57, 95–96, 124–25, 128,
197–98, 202, 210, 212, 220
West Florida Midwife Institute, 42

White House Conference on Child
Health and Protection, 1–3, 235
(n. 1)
Whitford, Grace, 34
Williams, J. Whitridge, 38–39
Works Progress Administration, 48